Eating Disorders

Eating Disorders

Edited by James Defoe

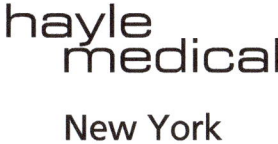

New York

Hayle Medical,
750 Third Avenue, 9ᵗʰ Floor,
New York, NY 10017, USA

Visit us on the World Wide Web at:
www.haylemedical.com

ISBN: 978-1-63241-493-9

Trademark Notice: Registered trademark of products or corporate names are used only for explanation and identification without intent to infringe.

Cataloging-in-Publication Data

Eating disorders / edited by James Defoe.
    p. cm.
Includes bibliographical references and index.
ISBN 978-1-63241-493-9
1. Eating disorders. I. Defoe, James.
RC552.E18 E28 2018
616.852 6--dc23

Table of Contents

Preface

Eating disorders are mental disorders which result in unnatural eating habits, like binge eating disorder or anorexia nervosa. These diseases result in deteriorated mental state and cause physical damage to the body of the patient. Usually the patients dealing with eating disorders also suffer from depression, anxiety and substance abuse. This book unfolds the innovative aspects of this field which will be crucial for the holistic understanding of the subject matter. It attempts to understand the varied types of eating disorders, their diagnosis and treatment. For someone with an interest and eye for detail, this book covers the most significant topics in this area.

A short introduction to every chapter is written below to provide an overview of the content of the book:

Chapter 1 - Eating habits that can cause psychological or physical problems are eating disorders. The causes for eating disorders can either be genetics or psychological and environmental factors. Diordered eating and ingestive behaviors are other themes that have been explored. This chapter will provide an integrated understanding of eating disorders; **Chapter 2 -** Eating disorders can be of various types like anorexia nervosa, bulimia nervosa, binge eating disorder and muscle dysmorphia. Anorexia nervosa is a psychological disorder which is defined by an extremely low body weight whereas binge eating disorder leads to uncontrollable eating. The major categories of eating disorders are dealt with great details in the chapter; **Chapter 3 -** Eating disorders can be diagnosed by using several diagnostic techniques like eating attitudes test, eating disorder inventory, SCOFF questionnaire, body attitudes questionnaire, body mass index, etc. Only a trained professional can take these tests. The aspects elucidated in this chapter are of vital importance, and provide a better understanding of eating disorders; **Chapter 4 -** Cognitive behavioral therapy is the therapy given to patients with eating disorders in order to alter or reduce their negative thoughts. Other treatments given to patients emphasize the social, biological, psychological and emotional harm caused by the disorder. Eating disorder is best understood in confluence with the major topics listed in the following chapter.

Finally, I would like to thank my fellow scholars who gave constructive feedback and my family members who supported me at every step.

Editor

Understanding Eating Disorders

Eating habits that can cause psychological or physical problems are eating disorders. The causes for eating disorders can either be genetics or psychological and environmental factors. Diordered eating and ingestive behaviors are other themes that have been explored. This chapter will provide an integrated understanding of eating disorders.

Eating Disorder

An eating disorder is a mental disorder defined by abnormal eating habits that negatively affect a person's physical or mental health. They include binge eating disorder where people eat a large amount in a short period of time, anorexia nervosa where people eat very little and thus have a low body weight, bulimia nervosa where people eat a lot and then try to rid themselves of the food, pica where people eat non-food items, rumination disorder where people regurgitate food, avoidant/restrictive food intake disorder where people have a lack of interest in food, and a group of other specified feeding or eating disorders. Anxiety disorders, depression, and substance abuse are common among people with eating disorders. These disorders do not include obesity.

The cause of eating disorders is not clear. Both biological and environmental factors appear to play a role. Cultural idealization of thinness is believed to contribute. Eating disorders affect about 12 percent of dancers. Those who have experienced sexual abuse are also more likely to develop eating disorders. Some disorders such as pica and rumination disorder occur more often in people with intellectual disabilities. Only one eating disorder can be diagnosed at a given time.

Treatment can be effective for many eating disorders. This typically involves counselling, a proper diet, a normal amount of exercise, and the reduction of efforts to eliminate food. Hospitalization is occasionally needed. Medications may be used to help with some of the associated symptoms. At five years about 70% of people with anorexia and 50% of people with bulimia recover. Recovery from binge eating disorder is less clear and estimated at 20% to 60%. Both anorexia and bulimia increase the risk of death.

In the developed world binge eating disorder affects about 1.6% of women and 0.8% of men in a given year. Anorexia affects about 0.4% and bulimia affects about 1.3% of young women in a given year. During the entire life up to 4% of women have anorexia, 2% have bulimia, and 2% have binge eating disorder. Anorexia and bulimia occur nearly ten times more often in females than males. Typically they begin in late childhood or early adulthood. Rates of other eating disorders are not clear. Rates of eating disorders appear to be lower in less developed countries.

Classification

Bulimia nervosa is a disorder characterized by binge eating and purging, as well as excessive evaluation of one's self-worth in terms of body weight or shape. Purging can include self-induced vomiting, over-exercising, and the use of diuretics, enemas, and laxatives. Anorexia nervosa is characterized by extreme food restriction and excessive weight loss, accompanied by the fear of being fat. The extreme weight loss often causes women and girls who have begun menstruating to stop having menstrual periods, a condition known as amenorrhea. Although amenorrhea was once a required criterion for the disorder, it is no longer required to meet criteria for anorexia nervosa due to its exclusive nature for sufferers who are male, post-menopause, or who do not menstruate for other reasons. The DSM-5 specifies two subtypes of anorexia nervosa—the restricting type and the binge/purge type. Those who suffer from the restricting type of anorexia nervosa restrict food intake and do not engage in binge eating, whereas those suffering from the binge/purge type lose control over their eating at least occasionally and may compensate for these binge episodes. The most notable difference between anorexia nervosa binge/purge type and bulimia nervosa is the body weight of the person. Those diagnosed with anorexia nervosa binge/purge type are underweight, while those with bulimia nervosa may have a body weight that falls within the range from normal to obese.

ICD and DSM

These eating disorders are specified as mental disorders in standard medical manuals, such as in the ICD-10, the DSM-5, or both.

- Anorexia nervosa (AN), characterized by lack of maintenance of a healthy body weight, an obsessive fear of gaining weight or refusal to do so, and an unrealistic perception, or non-recognition of the seriousness, of current low body weight. Anorexia can cause menstruation to stop, and often leads to bone loss, loss of skin integrity, etc. It greatly stresses the heart, increasing the risk of heart attacks and related heart problems. The risk of death is greatly increased in individuals with this disease. The most underlining factor researchers are starting to take notice of is that it may not just be a vanity, social, or media issue, but it could also be related to biological and or genetic components. The DSM-5 contains many changes that better represent patients with these conditions. The DSM-IV required amenorrhea (the absence of the menstrual cycle) to be present in order to diagnose a patient with anorexia. This is no longer a requirement in the DSM-5.

- Bulimia nervosa (BN), characterized by recurrent binge eating followed by compensatory behaviors such as purging (self-induced vomiting, eating to the point of vomiting, excessive use of laxatives/diuretics, or excessive exercise). Fasting and over-exercising may also be used as a method of purging following a binge.

- Muscle dysmorphia is characterized by appearance preoccupation that one's own body is too small, too skinny, insufficiently muscular, or insufficiently lean. Muscle dysmorphia affects mostly males.

- Binge Eating Disorder (BED), characterized by recurring binge eating at least once a week for over a period of 3 months while experiencing lack of control and guilt after overeating. The disorder can develop within individuals of a wide range of ages and socioeconomic classes.

- Other Specified Feeding or Eating Disorder (OSFED) is an eating or feeding disorder that does not meet full DSM-5 criteria for AN, BN, or BED. Examples of otherwise-specified eating disorders include individuals with atypical anorexia nervosa, who meet all criteria for AN except being underweight, despite substantial weight loss; atypical bulimia nervosa, who meet all criteria for BN except that bulimic behaviors are less frequent or have not been ongoing for long enough; purging disorder; and night eating syndrome.

Other

- Compulsive overeating (COE), in which individuals habitually graze on large quantities of food rather than binging, as would be typical of binge eating disorder.

- Prader-Willi syndrome

- Diabulimia, characterized by the deliberate manipulation of insulin levels by diabetics in an effort to control their weight.

- Food maintenance, characterized by a set of aberrant eating behaviors of children in foster care.

- Orthorexia nervosa, a term used by Steven Bratman to characterize an obsession with a "pure" diet, in which people develop an obsession with avoiding unhealthy foods to the point where it interferes with a person's life.

- Selective eating disorder, also called picky eating, is an extreme sensitivity to how something tastes. A person with SED may or may not be a supertaster.

- Drunkorexia, commonly characterized by purposely restricting food intake in order to reserve food calories for alcoholic calories, exercising excessively in order to burn calories consumed from drinking, and over-drinking alcohols in order to purge previously consumed food.

- Pregorexia, characterized by extreme dieting and over-exercising in order to control pregnancy weight gain. Undernutrition during pregnancy is associated with low birth weight, coronary heart disease, type 2 diabetes, stroke, hypertension, cardiovascular disease risk, and depression.

- Gourmand syndrome, a rare condition occurring after damage to the frontal lobe, resulting in an obsessive focus on fine foods.

Signs and Symptoms

Symptoms and complications vary according to the nature and severity of the eating disorder:

Possible Symptoms and Complications of Eating Disorders			
acne	xerosis	amenorrhoea	tooth loss, cavities
constipation	diarrhea	water retention and/or edema	lanugo
telogen effluvium	cardiac arrest	hypokalemia	death
osteoporosis	electrolyte imbalance	hyponatremia	brain atrophy
pellagra	scurvy	kidney failure	suicide

Some physical symptoms of eating disorders are weakness, fatigue, sensitivity to cold, reduced beard growth in men, reduction in waking erections, reduced libido, weight loss and failure of growth. Unexplained hoarseness may be a symptom of an underlying eating disorder, as the result of acid reflux, or entry of acidic gastric material into the laryngoesophageal tract. Patients who induce vomiting, such as those with anorexia nervosa, binge eating-purging type or those with purging-type bulimia nervosa are at risk for acid reflux. Polycystic ovary syndrome (PCOS) is the most common endocrine disorder to affect women. Though often associated with obesity it can occur in normal weight individuals. PCOS has been associated with binge eating and bulimic behavior. Other possible manifestations are dry lips, burning tongue, parotid gland swelling, and temporomandibular disorders.

Pro-ana Subculture

Pro-ana refers to the promotion of behaviors related to the eating disorder anorexia nervosa. Several websites promote eating disorders, and can provide a means for individuals to communicate in order to maintain eating disorders. Members of these websites typically feel that their eating disorder is the only aspect of a chaotic life that they can control. These websites are often interactive and have discussion boards where individuals can share strategies, ideas, and experiences, such as diet and exercise plans that achieve extremely low weights. A study comparing the personal web-blogs that were pro-eating disorder with those focused on recovery found that the pro-eating disorder blogs contained language reflecting lower cognitive processing, used a more closed-minded writing style, contained less emotional expression and fewer social references, and focused more on eating-related contents than did the recovery blogs.

Psychopathology

The psychopathology of eating disorders centers around body image disturbance, such as concerns with weight and shape; self-worth being too dependent on weight and shape; fear of gaining weight even when underweight; denial of how severe the symptoms are and a distortion in the way the body is experienced.

Causes

Many people with eating disorders suffer also from body dysmorphic disorder, altering the way a person sees themself. Studies have found that a high proportion of individuals diagnosed with body dysmorphic disorder also had some type of eating disorder, with 15% of individuals having either anorexia nervosa or bulimia nervosa. This link between body dysmorphic disorder and anorexia stems from the fact that both BDD and anorexia nervosa are characterized by a preoccupation with physical appearance and a distortion of body image. There are also many other possibilities such as environmental, social and interpersonal issues that could promote and sustain these illnesses.} Also, the media are oftentimes blamed for the rise in the incidence of eating disorders due to the fact that media images of idealized slim physical shape of people such as models and celebrities motivate or even force people to attempt to achieve slimness themselves. The media are accused of distorting reality, in the sense that people portrayed in the media are either naturally thin and thus unrepresentative of normality or unnaturally thin by forcing their bodies to look like the ideal image by putting excessive pressure on themselves to look a certain way. While past findings have described the causes of eating disorders as primarily psychological, environmental, and sociocultural, new studies have uncovered evidence that there is a prevalent genetic/heritable aspect of the causes of eating disorders.

Genetics

Numerous studies show a possible genetic predisposition toward eating disorders as a result of Mendelian inheritance. Twin studies have found a slight instances of genetic variance when considering the different criterion of both anorexia nervosa and bulimia nervosa as endophenotypes contributing to the disorders as a whole. A genetic link has been found on chromosome 1 in multiple family members of an individual with anorexia nervosa. An individual who is a first degree relative of someone who has or currently has an eating disorder is seven to twelve times more likely have an eating disorder themselves. Twin studies also show that at least a portion of the vulnerability to develop eating disorders can be inherited, and there is evidence to show that there is a genetic locus that shows susceptibility for developing anorexia nervosa. About 60% of eating disorder cases are attributable to biological and genetic components. Other cases are due to external reasons or developmental problems. There are also other neurobiological factors at play tied to emotional reactivity and impulsivity that could lead to binging and purging behaviors.

Epigenetics: Epigenetic mechanisms are means by which environmental effects alter gene expression via methods such as DNA methylation; these are independent of and do not alter the underlying DNA sequence. They are heritable, but also may occur throughout the lifespan, and are potentially reversible. Dysregulation of dopaminergic neurotransmission due to epigenetic mechanisms has been implicated in various eating disorders. One study has found that "epigenetic mechanisms may contribute to the known alterations of ANP homeostasis in women with eating disorders." Other candidate genes for epigenetic studies in eating disorders include leptin, pro-opiomelanocortin (POMC) and brain-derived neurotrophic factor (BDNF).

Psychological

Eating disorders are classified as Axis I disorders in the Diagnostic and Statistical Manual of Mental Health Disorders (DSM-IV) published by the American Psychiatric Association. There are various other psychological issues that may factor into eating disorders, some fulfill the criteria for a separate Axis I diagnosis or a personality disorder which is coded Axis II and thus are considered comorbid to the diagnosed eating disorder. Axis II disorders are subtyped into 3 "clusters": A, B and C. The causality between personality disorders and eating disorders has yet to be fully established. Some people have a previous disorder which may increase their vulnerability to developing an eating disorder. Some develop them afterwards. The severity and type of eating disorder symptoms have been shown to affect comorbidity. The DSM-IV should not be used by laypersons to diagnose themselves, even when used by professionals there has been considerable controversy over the diagnostic criteria used for various diagnoses, including eating disorders. There has been controversy over various editions of the DSM including the latest edition, DSM-V, due in May 2013.

Cognitive Attentional Bias Issues

Attentional bias may have an effect on eating disorders. Many studies have been performed to test this theory.

Comorbid Disorders	
Axis I	**Axis II**
depression	obsessive compulsive personality disorder
substance abuse, alcoholism	borderline personality disorder
anxiety disorders	narcissistic personality disorder
obsessive compulsive disorder	histrionic personality disorder
Attention-deficit hyperactivity disorder	avoidant personality disorder

Personality Traits

There are various childhood personality traits associated with the development of eating disorders. During adolescence these traits may become intensified due to a variety of physiological and cultural influences such as the hormonal changes associated with puberty, stress related to the approaching demands of maturity and socio-cultural influences and perceived expectations, especially in areas that concern body image. Eating disorders have been associated with a fragile sense of self and with disordered mentalization. Many personality traits have a genetic component and are highly heritable. Maladaptive levels of certain traits may be acquired as a result of anoxic or traumatic brain injury, neurodegenerative diseases such as Parkinson's disease, neurotoxicity such as lead exposure, bacterial infection such as Lyme disease or viral infection such as Toxoplasma gondii as well as hormonal influences. While studies are still continuing via the use of various imaging techniques such as fMRI; these traits have been shown to originate in various regions of the brain such as the amygdala and the prefrontal cortex. Disorders in the prefrontal cortex and the executive functioning system have been shown to affect eating behavior.

Celiac Disease

People with gastrointestinal disorders may be more risk of developing disordered eating practices than the general population, principally restrictive eating disturbances. An association of anorexia nervosa with celiac disease has been found. The role that gastrointestinal symptoms play in the development of eating disorders seems rather complex. Some authors report that unresolved symptoms prior to gastrointestinal disease diagnosis may create a food aversion in these persons, causing alterations to their eating patterns. Other authors report that greater symptoms throughout their diagnosis led to greater risk. It has been documented that some people with celiac disease, irritable bowel syndrome or inflammatory bowel disease who are not conscious about the importance of strictly following their diet, choose to consume their trigger foods to promote weight loss. On the other hand, individuals with good dietary management may develop anxiety, food aversion and eating disorders because of concerns around cross contamination of their foods. Some authors suggest that medical professionals should evaluate the presence of an unrecognized celiac disease in all people with eating disorder, especially if they present any gastrointestinal symptom (such as decreased appetite, abdominal pain, bloating, distension, vomiting, diarrhea or constipation), weight loss, or growth failure; and also routinely ask celiac patients about weight or body shape concerns, dieting or vomiting for weight control, to evaluate the possible presence of eating disorders, specially in women.

Environmental Influences

Child Maltreatment

Child abuse which encompasses physical, psychological and sexual abuse, as well as neglect has been shown to approximately triple the risk of an eating disorder. Sexual abuse appears to about double the risk of bulimia; however, the association is less clear for anorexia.

Social Isolation

Social isolation has been shown to have a deleterious effect on an individual's physical and emotional well-being. Those that are socially isolated have a higher mortality rate in general as compared to individuals that have established social relationships. This effect on mortality is markedly increased in those with pre-existing medical or psychiatric conditions, and has been especially noted in cases of coronary heart disease. "The magnitude of risk associated with social isolation is comparable with that of cigarette smoking and other major biomedical and psychosocial risk factors." (Brummett *et al.*)

Social isolation can be inherently stressful, depressing and anxiety-provoking. In an attempt to ameliorate these distressful feelings an individual may engage in emotional eating in which food serves as a source of comfort. The loneliness of social isolation and the inherent stressors thus associated have been implicated as triggering factors in binge eating as well.

Waller, Kennerley and Ohanian (2007) argued that both bingeing–vomiting and restriction are emotion suppression strategies, but they are just utilized at different times. For example, restriction is used to pre-empt any emotion activation, while bingeing–vomiting is used after an emotion has been activated.

Parental Influence

Parental influence has been shown to be an intrinsic component in the development of eating behaviors of children. This influence is manifested and shaped by a variety of diverse factors such as familial genetic predisposition, dietary choices as dictated by cultural or ethnic preferences, the parents' own body shape and eating patterns, the degree of involvement and expectations of their children's eating behavior as well as the interpersonal relationship of parent and child. This is in addition to the general psychosocial climate of the home and the presence or absence of a nurturing stable environment. It has been shown that maladaptive parental behavior has an important role in the development of eating disorders. As to the more subtle aspects of parental influence, it has been shown that eating patterns are established in early childhood and that children should be allowed to decide when their appetite is satisfied as early as the age of two. A direct link has been shown between obesity and parental pressure to eat more.

Coercive tactics in regard to diet have not been proven to be efficacious in controlling a child's eating behavior. Affection and attention have been shown to affect the degree of a child's finickiness and their acceptance of a more varied diet.

Hilde Bruch, a pioneer in the field of studying eating disorders, asserts that anorexia nervosa often occurs in girls who are high achievers, obedient, and always trying to please their parents. Their parents have a tendency to be over-controlling and fail to encourage the expression of emotions, inhibiting daughters from accepting their own feelings and desires. Adolescent females in these overbearing families lack the ability to be independent from their families, yet realize the need to, often resulting in rebellion. Controlling their food intake may make them feel better, as it provides them with a sense of control.

Peer Pressure

In various studies such as one conducted by The McKnight Investigators, peer pressure was shown to be a significant contributor to body image concerns and attitudes toward eating among subjects in their teens and early twenties.

Eleanor Mackey and co-author, Annette M. La Greca of the University of Miami, studied 236 teen girls from public high schools in southeast Florida. "Teen girls' concerns about their own weight, about how they appear to others and their perceptions that their peers want them to be thin are significantly related to weight-control behavior", says psychologist Eleanor Mackey of the Children's National Medical Center in Washington and lead author of the study. "Those are really important."

According to one study, 40% of 9- and 10-year-old girls are already trying to lose weight. Such dieting is reported to be influenced by peer behavior, with many of those individuals on a diet reporting that their friends also were dieting. The number of friends dieting and the number of friends who pressured them to diet also played a significant role in their own choices.

Elite athletes have a significantly higher rate in eating disorders. Female athletes in sports such as gymnastics, ballet, diving, etc. are found to be at the highest risk among all athletes. Women are more likely than men to acquire an eating disorder between the ages of 13–30. 0–15% of those with bulimia and anorexia are men.

Cultural Pressure

There is a cultural emphasis on thinness which is especially pervasive in western society. There is an unrealistic stereotype of what constitutes beauty and the ideal body type as portrayed by the media, fashion and entertainment industries. "The cultural pressure on men and women to be 'perfect' is an important predisposing factor for the development of eating disorders". Further, when women of all races base their evaluation of their self upon what is considered the culturally ideal body, the incidence of eating disorders increases. Eating disorders are becoming more prevalent in non-Western countries where thinness is not seen as the ideal, showing that social and cultural pressures are not the only causes of eating disorders. For example, observations of anorexia in all of the non-Western regions of the world point to the disorder not being "culture-bound" as once thought. However, studies on rates of bulimia suggest that it might be culturally bound. In non-Western countries, bulimia is less prevalent than anorexia, but these non-Western countries where it is observed can be said to have probably or definitely been influenced or exposed to Western culture and ideology.

Socioeconomic status (SES) has been viewed as a risk factor for eating disorders, presuming that possessing more resources allows for an individual to actively choose to diet and reduce body weight. Some studies have also shown a relationship between increasing body dissatisfaction with increasing SES. However, once high socioeconomic status has been achieved, this relationship weakens and, in some cases, no longer exists.

The media plays a major role in the way in which people view themselves. Countless magazine ads and commercials depict thin celebrities like Lindsay Lohan, Nicole Richie, Victoria Beckham and Mary Kate Olsen, who appear to gain nothing but attention from their looks. Society has taught people that being accepted by others is necessary at all costs. Unfortunately this has led to the belief that in order to fit in one must look a certain way. Televised beauty competitions such as the Miss America Competition contribute to the idea of what it means to be beautiful because competitors are evaluated on the basis of their opinion.

In addition to socioeconomic status being considered a cultural risk factor so is the world of sports. Athletes and eating disorders tend to go hand in hand, especially the sports where weight is a competitive factor. Gymnastics, horse back riding, wrestling, body building, and dancing are just a few that fall into this category of weight dependent sports. Eating disorders among individuals that participate in competitive activities, especially women, often lead to having physical and biological changes related to their weight that often mimic prepubescent stages. Oftentimes as women's bodies change they lose their competitive edge which leads them to taking extreme measures to maintain their younger body shape. Men often struggle with binge eating followed by excessive exercise while focusing on building muscle rather than losing fat, but this goal of gaining muscle is just as much an eating disorder as obsessing over thinness. The following statistics taken from Susan Nolen-Hoeksema's book, *(ab)normal psychology*, shows the estimated percentage of athletes that struggle with eating disorders based on the category of sport.

- Aesthetic sports (dance, figure skating, gymnastics) – 35%

- Weight dependent sports (judo, wrestling) – 29%

- Endurance sports (cycling, swimming, running) – 20%

- Technical sports (golf, high jumping) – 14%

- Ball game sports (volleyball, soccer) – 12%

Although most of these athletes develop eating disorders to keep their competitive edge, others use exercise as a way to maintain their weight and figure. This is just as serious as regulating food intake for competition. Even though there is mixed evidence showing at what point athletes are challenged with eating disorders, studies show that regardless of competition level all athletes are at higher risk for developing eating disorders that non-athletes, especially those that participate in sports where thinness is a factor.

Pressure from society is also seen within the homosexual community. Homosexual men are at greater risk of eating disorder symptoms than heterosexual men. Within the gay culture, muscularity gives the advantages of both social and sexual desirability and also power. These pressures and ideas that another homosexual male may desire a mate who is thinner or muscular can possibly lead to eating disorders. The higher eating disorder symptom score reported, the more concern about how others perceive them and the more frequent and excessive exercise sessions occur. High levels of body dissatisfaction are also linked to external motivation to working out and old age; however, having a thin and muscular body occurs within younger homosexual males than older.

It is important to realize some of the limitations and challenges of many studies that try to examine the roles of culture, ethnicity, and SES. For starters, most of the cross-cultural studies use definitions from the DSM-IV-TR, which has been criticized as reflecting a Western cultural bias. Thus, assessments and questionnaires may not be constructed to detect some of the cultural differences associated with different disorders. Also, when looking at individuals in areas potentially influenced by Western culture, few studies have attempted to measure how much an individual has adopted the mainstream culture or retained the traditional cultural values of the area. Lastly, the majority of the cross-cultural studies on eating disorders and body image disturbances occurred in Western nations and not in the countries or regions being examined.

While there are many influences to how an individual processes their body image, the media does play a major role. Along with the media, parental influence, peer influence, and self-efficacy beliefs also play a large role in an individual's view of themselves. The way the media presents images can have a lasting effect on an individual's perception of their body image. Eating disorders are a worldwide issue and while women are more likely to be affected by an eating disorder it still affects both genders (Schwitzer 2012). The media influences eating disorders whether shown in a positive or negative light, it then has a responsibility to use caution when promoting images that projects an ideal that many turn to eating disorders to attain.

To try to address unhealthy body image in the fashion world, in 2015, France passed a law requiring models to be declared healthy by a doctor to participate in fashion shows. It also requires retouched images to be marked as such in magazines.

There is a relationship between "thin ideal" social media content and body dissatisfaction and eating disorders among young adult women, especially in the Western hemisphere. New research points to an "internalization" of distorted images online, as well as negative comparisons among young adult women. Most studies have been based in the U.S, the U.K, and Australia, these are places where the thin ideal is strong among women, as well as the strive for the "perfect" body.

In addition to mere media exposure, there is an online "pro-eating disorder" community. Through personal blogs and Twitter, this community promotes eating disorders as a "lifestyle", and continuously posts pictures of emaciated bodies, and tips on how to stay thin. The hashtag "#proana" (pro-anorexia), is a product of this community, as well as images promoting weight loss, tagged with the term "thinspiration". According to social comparison theory, young women have a tendency to compare their appearance to others, which can result in a negative view of their own bodies and altering of eating behaviors, that in turn can develop disordered eating behaviors.

When body parts are isolated and displayed in the media as objects to be looked at, it is called objectification, and women are affected most by this phenomenon. Objectification increases self-objectification, where women judge their own body parts as a mean of praise and pleasure for others. There is a significant link between self-objectification, body dissatisfaction, and disordered eating, as the beauty ideal is altered through social media.

Mechanisms

- Biochemical: Eating behavior is a complex process controlled by the neuroendocrine system, of which the Hypothalamus-pituitary-adrenal-axis (HPA axis) is a major component. Dysregulation of the HPA axis has been associated with eating disorders, such as irregularities in the manufacture, amount or transmission of certain neurotransmitters, hormones or neuropeptides and amino acids such as homocysteine, elevated levels of which are found in AN and BN as well as depression.

  o Serotonin: a neurotransmitter involved in depression also has an inhibitory effect on eating behavior.

  o Norepinephrine is both a neurotransmitter and a hormone; abnormalities in either capacity may affect eating behavior.

  o Dopamine: which in addition to being a precursor of norepinephrine and epinephrine is also a neurotransmitter which regulates the rewarding property of food.

  o Neuropeptide Y also known as NPY is a hormone that encourages eating and decreases metabolic rate. Blood levels of NPY are elevated in patients with anorexia nervosa, and studies have shown that injection of this hormone into the brain of rats with restricted food intake increases their time spent running on a wheel. Normally the hormone stimulates eating in healthy patients, but under conditions of starvation it increases their activity rate, probably to increase the chance of finding food. The increased levels of NPY in the blood of patients with eating disorders can in some ways explain the instances of extreme over-exercising found in most anorexia nervosa patients.

- Leptin and ghrelin: leptin is a hormone produced primarily by the fat cells in the body; it has an inhibitory effect on appetite by inducing a feeling of satiety. Ghrelin is an appetite inducing hormone produced in the stomach and the upper portion of the small intestine. Circulating levels of both hormones are an important factor in weight control. While often associated with obesity, both hormones and their respective effects have been implicated in the pathophysiology of anorexia nervosa and bulimia nervosa. Leptin can also be used to distinguish between constitutional thinness found in a healthy person with a low BMI and an individual with anorexia nervosa.

- Gut bacteria and immune system: studies have shown that a majority of patients with anorexia and bulimia nervosa have elevated levels of autoantibodies that affect hormones and neuropeptides that regulate appetite control and the stress response. There may be a direct correlation between autoantibody levels and associated psychological traits. Later study revealed that autoantibodies reactive with alpha-MSH are, in fact, generated against ClpB, a protein produced by certain gut bacteria e.g. Escherichia coli. ClpB protein was identified as a conformational antigen-mimetic of alpha-MSH. In patients with eating disorders plasma levels of anti-ClpB IgG and IgM correalated with patients' psychological traits

- Infection: PANDAS, is an abbreviation for Pediatric Autoimmune Neuropsychiatric Disorders Associated with Streptococcal Infections. Children with PANDAS "have obsessive-compulsive disorder (OCD) and/or tic disorders such as Tourette syndrome, and in whom symptoms worsen following infections such as "strep throat" and scarlet fever". (NIMH) There is a possibility that PANDAS may be a precipitating factor in the development of anorexia nervosa in some cases, (PANDAS AN).

- Lesions: studies have shown that lesions to the right frontal lobe or temporal lobe can cause the pathological symptoms of an eating disorder.

- Tumors: tumors in various regions of the brain have been implicated in the development of abnormal eating patterns.

- Brain calcification: a study highlights a case in which prior calcification of the right thalamus may have contributed to development of anorexia nervosa.

- somatosensory homunculus: is the representation of the body located in the somatosensory cortex, first described by renowned neurosurgeon Wilder Penfield. The illustration was originally termed "Penfield's Homunculus", homunculus meaning little man. "In normal development this representation should adapt as the body goes through its pubertal growth spurt. However, in AN it is hypothesized that there is a lack of plasticity in this area, which may result in impairments of sensory processing and distortion of body image". (Bryan Lask, also proposed by VS Ramachandran)

- Obstetric complications: There have been studies done which show maternal smoking, obstetric and perinatal complications such as maternal anemia, very pre-term birth (less than 32 weeks), being born small for gestational age, neonatal cardiac problems, preeclampsia, placental infarction and sustaining a cephalhematoma at birth increase the risk factor for developing either anorexia nervosa or bulimia nervosa. Some of this developmental risk as in the case of placental infarction, maternal anemia and cardiac problems may cause intra-uterine hypoxia, umbilical cord occlusion or cord prolapse may cause ischemia, resulting in cerebral injury, the prefrontal cortex in the fetus and neonate is highly susceptible to damage as a result of oxygen deprivation which has been shown to contribute to executive dysfunction, ADHD, and may affect personality traits associated with both eating disorders and comorbid disorders such as impulsivity, mental rigidity and obsessionality. The problem of perinatal brain injury, in terms of the costs to society and to the affected individuals and their families, is extraordinary. (Yafeng Dong, PhD)

- Symptom of starvation: Evidence suggests that the symptoms of eating disorders are actually symptoms of the starvation itself, not of a mental disorder. In a study involving thirty-six healthy young men that were subjected to semi-starvation, the men soon began displaying symptoms commonly found in patients with eating disorders. In this study, the healthy men ate approximately half of what they had become accustomed to eating and soon began developing symptoms and thought patterns (preoccupation with food and eating, ritualistic eating, impaired cognitive ability, other physiological changes such as decreased body temperature) that are characteristic symptoms of anorexia nervosa. The men used in the study also developed hoarding and obsessive collecting behaviors, even though they had no use for the items, which revealed a possible connection between eating disorders and obsessive compulsive disorder.

Diagnosis

The initial diagnosis should be made by a competent medical professional. "The medical history is the most powerful tool for diagnosing eating disorders"(American Family Physician). There are many medical disorders that mimic eating disorders and comorbid psychiatric disorders. All organic causes should be ruled out prior to a diagnosis of an eating disorder or any other psychiatric disorder. In the past 30 years eating disorders have become increasingly conspicuous and it is uncertain whether the changes in presentation reflect a true increase. Anorexia nervosa and bulimia nervosa are the most clearly defined subgroups of a wider range of eating disorders. Many patients present with subthreshold expressions of the two main diagnoses: others with different patterns and symptoms.

Medical

The diagnostic workup typically includes complete medical and psychosocial history and follows a rational and formulaic approach to the diagnosis. Neuroimaging using fMRI, MRI, PET and SPECT scans have been used to detect cases in which a lesion, tumor or other organic condition has been either the sole causative or contributory factor in an eating disorder. "Right frontal intracerebral lesions with their close relationship to the limbic system could be causative for eating disorders, we therefore recommend performing a cranial MRI in all patients with suspected eating disorders" (Trummer M *et al.* 2002), "intracranial pathology should also be considered however certain is the diagnosis of early-onset anorexia nervosa. Second, neuroimaging plays an important part in diagnosing early-onset anorexia nervosa, both from a clinical and a research prospective". (O'Brien *et al.* 2001).

Psychological

Eating Disorder Specific Psychometric Tests	
Eating Attitudes Test	SCOFF questionnaire
Body Attitudes Test	Body Attitudes Questionnaire
Eating Disorder Inventory	Eating Disorder Examination Interview

After ruling out organic causes and the initial diagnosis of an eating disorder being made by a medical professional, a trained mental health professional aids in the assessment and treatment of the underlying psychological components of the eating disorder and any comorbid psychological conditions. The clinician conducts a clinical interview and may employ various psychometric tests. Some are general in nature while others were devised specifically for use in the assessment of eating disorders. Some of the general tests that may be used are the Hamilton Depression Rating Scale and the Beck Depression Inventory. longitudinal research showed that there is an increase in chance that a young adult female would develop bulimia due to their current psychological pressure and as the person ages and matures, their emotional problems change or are resolved and then the symptoms decline.

Differential Diagnoses

There are multiple medical conditions which may be misdiagnosed as a primary psychiatric disorder, complicating or delaying treatment. These may have a synergistic effect on conditions which mimic an eating disorder or on a properly diagnosed eating disorder.

- Lyme disease which is known as the "great imitator", as it may present as a variety of psychiatric or neurological disorders including anorexia nervosa.

- Gastrointestinal diseases, such as celiac disease, Crohn's disease, peptic ulcer, eosinophilic esophagitis or non-celiac gluten sensitivity, among others. Celiac disease is also known as the "great imitator", because it may involve several organs and cause an extensive variety of non-gastrointestinal symptoms, such as psychiatric and neurological disorders, including anorexia nervosa.

- Addison's Disease is a disorder of the adrenal cortex which results in decreased hormonal production. Addison's disease, even in subclinical form may mimic many of the symptoms of anorexia nervosa.

- Gastric adenocarcinoma is one of the most common forms of cancer in the world. Complications due to this condition have been misdiagnosed as an eating disorder.

- Hypothyroidism, hyperthyroidism, hypoparathyroidism and hyperparathyroidism may mimic some of the symptoms of, can occur concurrently with, be masked by or exacerbate an eating disorder.

- Toxoplasma seropositivity: even in the absence of symptomatic toxoplasmosis, toxoplasma gondii exposure has been linked to changes in human behavior and psychiatric disorders including those comorbid with eating disorders such as depression. In reported case studies the response to antidepressant treatment improved only after adequate treatment for toxoplasma.

- Neurosyphilis: It is estimated that there may be up to one million cases of untreated syphilis in the US alone. "The disease can present with psychiatric symptoms alone, psychiatric symptoms that can mimic any other psychiatric illness". Many of the manifestations may appear atypical. Up to 1.3% of short term psychiatric admissions may be attributable to neurosyphilis, with a much higher rate in the general psychiatric population. (Ritchie, M Perdigao J,)

- Dysautonomia: a wide variety of autonomic nervous system (ANS) disorders may cause a wide variety of psychiatric symptoms including anxiety, panic attacks and depression. Dysautonomia usually involves failure of sympathetic or parasympathetic components of the ANS system but may also include excessive ANS activity. Dysautonomia can occur in conditions such as diabetes and alcoholism.

Psychological disorders which may be confused with an eating disorder, or be co-morbid with one:

- Emetophobia is an anxiety disorder characterized by an intense fear of vomiting. A person so afflicted may develop rigorous standards of food hygiene, such as not touching food with their hands. They may become socially withdrawn to avoid situations which in their perception may make them vomit. Many who suffer from emetophobia are diagnosed with anorexia or self-starvation. In severe cases of emetophobia they may drastically reduce their food intake.

- Phagophobia is an anxiety disorder characterized by a fear of eating, it is usually initiated by an adverse experience while eating such as choking or vomiting. Persons with this disorder may present with complaints of pain while swallowing.

- Body dysmorphic disorder (BDD) is listed as a somatoform disorder that affects up to 2% of the population. BDD is characterized by excessive rumination over an actual or perceived physical flaw. BDD has been diagnosed equally among men and women. While BDD has been misdiagnosed as anorexia nervosa, it also occurs comorbidly in 39% of eating disorder cases. BDD is a chronic and debilitating condition which may lead to social isolation, major depression and suicidal ideation and attempts. Neuroimaging studies to measure response to facial recognition have shown activity predominately in the left hemisphere in the left lateral prefrontal cortex, lateral temporal lobe and left parietal lobe showing hemispheric imbalance in information processing. There is a reported case of the development of BDD in a 21-year-old male following an inflammatory brain process. Neuroimaging showed the presence of a new atrophy in the frontotemporal region.

Prevention

Prevention aims to promote a healthy development before the occurrence of eating disorders. It also intends early identification of an eating disorder before it is too late to treat. Children as young as ages 5–7 are aware of the cultural messages regarding body image and dieting. Prevention comes in bringing these issues to the light. The following topics can be discussed with young children (as well as teens and young adults).

- Emotional Bites: a simple way to discuss emotional eating is to ask children about why they might eat besides being hungry. Talk about more effective ways to cope with emotions, emphasizing the value of sharing feelings with a trusted adult.

- Say No to Teasing: another concept is to emphasize that it is wrong to say hurtful things about other people's body sizes.

- Body Talk: emphasize the importance of listening to one's body. That is, eating when you are hungry (not starving) and stopping when you are satisfied (not stuffed). Children intuitively grasp these concepts.

- Fitness Comes in All Sizes: educate children about the genetics of body size and the normal changes occurring in the body. Discuss their fears and hopes about growing bigger. Focus on fitness and a balanced diet.

Internet and modern technologies provide new opportunities for prevention. On-line programs have the potential to increase the use of prevention programs. The development and practice of prevention programs via on-line sources make it possible to reach a wide range of people at minimal cost. Such an approach can also make prevention programs to be sustainable.

Treatment

Treatment varies according to type and severity of eating disorder, and usually more than one treatment option is utilized. There is no well-established treatment for eating disorders, meaning that current views about treatment are based mainly on clinical experience. Family doctors play an important role in early treatment of people with eating disorders by encouraging those who are also reluctant to see a psychiatrist. Treatment can take place in a variety of different settings such as community programs, hospitals, day programs, and groups. The American Psychiatric Association (APA) recommends a team approach to treatment of eating disorders. The members of the team are usually a psychiatrist, therapist, and registered dietitian, but other clinicians may be included.

That said, some treatment methods are:

- Cognitive behavioral therapy (CBT), which postulates that an individual's feelings and behaviors are caused by their own thoughts instead of external stimuli such as other people, situations or events; the idea is to change how a person thinks and reacts to a situation even if the situation itself does not change.

  o Acceptance and commitment therapy: a type of CBT

  o Cognitive Remediation Therapy (CRT), a set of cognitive drills or compensatory interventions designed to enhance cognitive functioning.

- Dialectical behavior therapy

- Family therapy including "conjoint family therapy" (CFT), "separated family therapy" (SFT) and Maudsley Family Therapy.

- Behavioral therapy: focuses on gaining control and changing unwanted behaviors.

- Interpersonal psychotherapy (IPT)

- Cognitive Emotional Behaviour Therapy (CEBT)

- Music Therapy

- Recreation Therapy

- Art therapy

- Nutrition counseling and Medical nutrition therapy

- Medication: Orlistat is used in obesity treatment. Olanzapine seems to promote weight gain as well as the ability to ameliorate obsessional behaviors concerning weight gain. zinc supplements have been shown to be helpful, and cortisol is also being investigated.

- Self-help and guided self-help have been shown to be helpful in AN, BN and BED; this includes support groups and self-help groups such as Eating Disorders Anonymous and Overeaters Anonymous.

- Psychoanalysis

- Inpatient care

There are few studies on the cost-effectiveness of the various treatments. Treatment can be expensive; due to limitations in health care coverage, people hospitalized with anorexia nervosa may be discharged while still underweight, resulting in relapse and rehospitalization.

For children with anorexia, the only well-established treatment is the family treatment-behavior. For other eating disorders in children, however, there is no well-established treatments, though family treatment-behavior has been used in treating bulimia.

Outcomes

Outcome estimates are complicated by non-uniform criteria used by various studies, but for anorexia nervosa, bulimia nervosa, and binge eating disorder, there seems to be general agreement that full recovery rates are in the 50% to 85% range, with larger proportions of people experiencing at least partial remission. The outcomes of eating disorders (ED) vary among the cases. For many, it can be a lifelong struggle or it can be overcome within months. In the United States, twenty million women and ten million men have an eating disorders at least once in their lifetime. The mortality rate for those with anorexia nervosa is 5.4 per 1000 individuals per year. Roughly 1.3 deaths were due to suicide. A person who is or had been in an inpatient setting had a rate of 4.6 deaths per 1000. Of individuals with bulimia nervosa about 2 persons per 1000 persons die per year and among those with EDNOS about 3.3 per 1000 people die per year.

- Miscarriages: Pregnant women with a Binge Eating Disorder have shown to have a greater chance of having a miscarriage compared to pregnant women with any other eating disorders. According to a study done, out of a group of pregnant women being evaluated, 46.7% of the pregnancies ended with a miscarriage in women that were diagnosed with BED, with 23.0% in the control. In the same study, 21.4% of women diagnosed with Bulimia Nervosa had their pregnancies end with miscarriages and only 17.7% of the controls.

- Relapse: An individual who is in remission from BN and EDNOS (Eating Disorder Not Otherwise Specified) is at a high risk of falling back into the habit of self-harming themselves. Factors such as high stress regarding their job, pressures from society, as well as other occurrences that inflict stress on a person, can push a person back to what they feel will ease the pain. A study tracked a group of selected people that were either diagnosed with BN or EDNOS for 60 months. After the 60 months were complete, the researchers recorded whether or not the patients were suffering from a relapse. The results found that the probability of a person previously diagnosed with EDNOS had a 41% chance of relapsing; a person with BN had a 47% chance.

- Attachment insecurity: People who are showing signs of attachment anxiety will most likely have trouble communicating their emotional status as well as having trouble seeking effective social support. Signs that a person has adopted this symptom include not showing recognition to their caregiver or when he/she is feeling pain. In a clinical sample, it is clear that at the pretreatment step of a patient's recovery, more severe eating disorder symptoms directly corresponds to higher attachment anxiety. The more this symptom increases, the more difficult it is to achieve eating disorder reduction prior to treatment.

Anorexia Nervosa symptoms include the increasing chance of getting osteoporosis. This disease causes the bones of an individual to become brittle, weak, and low in density. Thinning of the hair as well as dry hair and skin is also very common. The muscles of the heart will also start to change if no treatment is inflicted on the patient. This causes the heart to have an abnormally slow heart rate along with low blood pressure. Heart failure becomes a major consideration when this begins to occur. Muscles throughout the body begin to lose their strength. This will cause the individual to begin feeling faint, drowsy, and weak. Along with these symptoms, the body will begin to grow a layer of hair called lanugo. The human body does this in response to the lack of heat and insulation due to the low percentage of body fat.

Bulimia nervosa symptoms include heart problems like an irregular heartbeat that can lead to heart failure and death may occur. This occurs because of the electrolyte imbalance that is a result of the constant binge and purge process. The probability of a gastric rupture increases. A gastric rupture is when there is a sudden rupture of the stomach lining that can be fatal.The acids that are contained in the vomit can cause a rupture in the esophagus as well as tooth decay. As a result, to laxative abuse, irregular bowel movements may occur along with constipation. Sores along the lining of the stomach called peptic ulcers begin to appear and the chance of developing pancreatitis increases.

Binge eating symptoms include high blood pressure, which can cause heart disease if it is not treated. Many patients recognize an increase in the levels of cholesterol. The chance of being diagnosed with gallbladder disease increases, which affects an individual's digestive tract.

Epidemiology

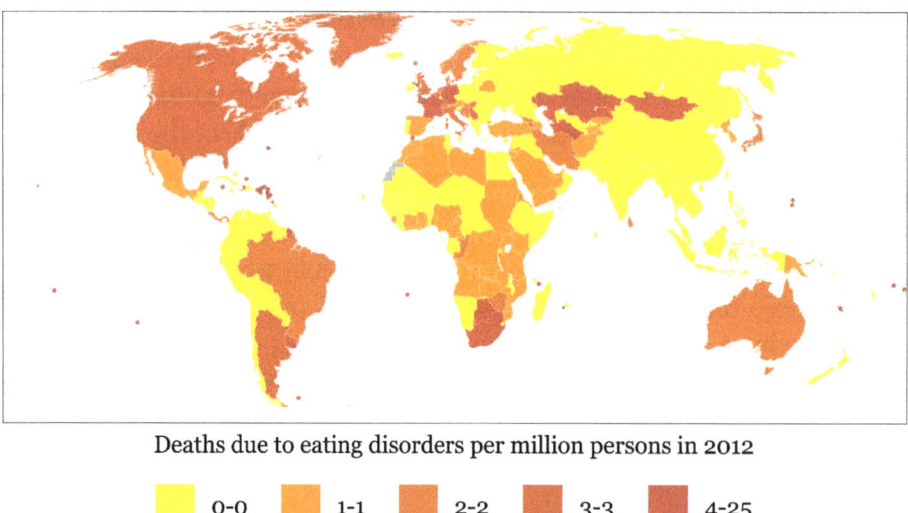

Deaths due to eating disorders per million persons in 2012

| | 0-0 | | 1-1 | | 2-2 | | 3-3 | | 4-25 |

Eating disorders result in about 7,000 deaths a year as of 2010, making them the mental illnesses with the highest mortality rate.

One study in the United States found a higher rate in college students who are transgender.

Economics

- Total costs in USA for hospital stays involving eating disorders rose from $165 million in

1999–2000 to $277 million in 2008–2009; this was a 68% increase. The mean cost per discharge of a person with an eating disorder rose by 29% over the decade, from $7,300 to $9,400.

- Over the decade, hospitalizations involving eating disorders increased among all age groups. The greatest increases occurred among those 45 to 65 years of age (an 88% increase), followed by hospitalizations among people younger than 12 years of age (a 72% increase).

- The majority of eating disorder inpatients were female. During 2008–2009, 88% of cases involved females, and 12% were males. The report also showed a 53% increase in hospitalizations for males with a principal diagnosis of an eating disorder, from 10% to 12% over the decade.

Eating Disorders and Memory

Many memory impairments exist as a result from or cause of eating disorders. Eating Disorders (ED) are characterized by abnormal and disturbed eating patterns that affect the lives of the individuals who worry about their weight to the extreme. These abnormal eating patterns involve either inadequate or excessive food intake, affecting the individual's physical and mental health.

In regard to mental health, individuals with eating disorders appear to have *memory impairments* in executive functioning, visual-spatial ability, divided and sustained attention, verbal functioning, learning, and memory. Some memory impairments found in individuals with ED, are due to nutritional deficiencies, as well as various cognitive and attentional biases. Neurobiological differences have been found in individuals with ED compared to healthy individuals, and these differences are reflected in specific memory impairments. There are certain treatments and effects of treatments, aimed at these ED-specific memory impairments. Animal research and areas of future research in relation to ED and memory, are also integral to understanding the effects of ED on memory. There are three particular diagnoses of eating disorders that have been linked to memory impairments: Anorexia Nervosa (AN), Bulimia Nervosa (BN), and Binge Eating Disorder (BED).

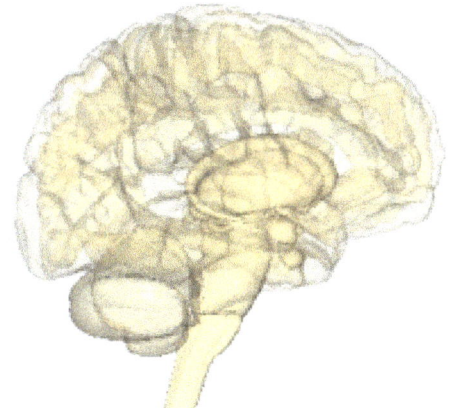

Many areas of the brain are affected by eating disorders, and this is reflected in memory performance.

Memory Impairments

Memory Biases

Individuals with eating disorders show increased tendencies to direct their attention towards irregular eating-related thought processing and attentional bias, compared to non-ED individuals. Studies have suggested a strong link between eating disorders and information processing such as attention and memory. All types of eating disorders (bulimia nervosa, anorexia nervosa, obesity and EDNOS) consistently display attentional biases towards disorder-related stimuli specific to their ED. Examples of disorder-related stimuli include food, shape, weight and size. This heightened attention to disorder-related stimuli leads to higher levels of encoding, consolidation and retrieval of this information, acting as a potential cause for the mental maintenance of the disorder(s).

Individuals with eating disorders display several memory and attentional biases to food, shape, weight and size. Specific memory biases include:

- Directed-forgetting: individuals with eating disorders, particularly anorexia nervosa, display more difficulty in forgetting information or cues related to body, shape and food than those without eating disorders. This leads to greater availability of such memories, facilitating the maintenance of the eating disorder.

- Schema-related: display maladaptive perceptions of food, shape, weight and self that lead to obsessive attention on and enhanced memory for these items, leading to maintaining the eating disorder thought and eating behaviour. Memories for these items are more easily encoded and retrieved compared to other information. Most of the research in this area has been on individuals with anorexia nervosa. Cued recall tasks, recognition tasks and Stroop task tests are used to study these effects. Some studies have shown contradictory results to ED individuals' heightened attention and enhanced memory, however the difference could be attributed to an anxiety-induced response and avoidance behaviour. This could cause impairments in the individuals' ability to remember the information learned, and suggests that more research needs to be done in this area to better understand the relationship between schema-related biases and ED's.

- Selective memory bias: studies have been done on individuals with bulimia nervosa, suggesting selective memory bias exists for positive and negative weight-related items compared to emotional items. Biases towards food-related items were also found, a common finding in individuals with depression.

Explicit Memory

Anorexia Nervosa (AN)

Patients with AN show a strong explicit memory bias towards anorexia-related words. In one study, participants (AN group compared to a control group) were presented with a list of words divided into four categories: positive, negative, neutral and anorexia-related. They were then tested explicitly with cued recall and it was found that the AN participants better favored the anorexia-related words, showing a *schema-related memory bias*. Participants were also tested implicitly with word stem completion tests, but no implicit bias was found.

In another study, AN participants were found to have less ability to concentrate in the presence of explicit distractors, as well as to have a conscious cognitive bias towards illness-related words. These explicit biases were associated with longer duration of the illness. A different study characterized AN patients as having trouble integrating positive and negative experiences and that the length of the illness also affected these symptoms and reinforced these impairments. The results of these studies suggest that there are clear differences in the explicit cognitive processing of stimuli between AN individuals and healthy controls and that length of the illness can affect the extent of these memory biases.

A different study showed that currently ill AN patients had problems with immediate and delayed verbal recall; these disadvantages were also found in weight-restored AN individuals. There was no difference between healthy controls and AN patients in working memory, just memory function. This study demonstrates that there are not only memory biases found in AN individuals, but memory impairments as well.

Autobiographical memory deficits have been found in individuals with AN. One study found that AN patients with a history of sexual abuse had impairments in their autobiographical memory characterized by their increased general memory recall. Another study found that anorexic patients are characterized by an over-generalization of both positive and negative autobiographical memories, which positively correlates with the duration of the illness. The impairment of both positive and negative memories suggests a general impairment in the access to emotional memories, therefore anorexic patients are more prone to suppress or control not only negative but also positive affect. One hypothesis suggests that these more general memories are what allow these patients to reduce the impact of a negative event.

Bulimia Nervosa (BN)

In one study, participants (BN and healthy controls) were exposed to television commercials that were neutral, food-related or body-related. Recall and recognition tests were carried out to test for an explicit memory bias. When compared to healthy controls, BN patients had less recall and recognition for body-related stimuli. This suggests that BN individuals avoid encoding/processing stimuli related to body image and have a *selective memory bias*.

Binge Eating Disorder (BED)

Obese individuals with binge eating disorder have been compared with obese controls to see if there are different explicit memory biases between these two groups of people. It was found that both groups showed a bias towards negative words, but individuals with BED retrieved positive words less often. This demonstrates an explicit memory bias in which individuals with BED avoid encoding or pay less attention to positive words and focus their conscious attention almost exclusively on negative words. This is similar to the *selective memory bias* mentioned above.

Implicit Memory

It was once thought that individuals with eating disorders had different implicit memory biases and attitudes towards food, depending on the type of eating disorder. BED was associated with positive evaluation of food and anorexia and bulimia were associated with negative evaluation of food. This turns out to not be the case. There were no implicit differences in affective attitudes towards foods between high and low-restraint eaters. This suggests that regardless of the type of eating disorder, individuals with eating disorders view food in similar ways and have similar implicit attitudes towards food.

Focusing on obesity, it has been found that obese individuals have more negative attitudes towards high-fat foods than a normal weight control group. It has also been found that children, particularly obese children, were faster at pushing a positive key than a negative key for food. These different attitudes towards food at different ages could represent different stages in development of obesity. Future research could be done to explore these effects found in obesity and determine if similar effects are seen in individuals with binge eating disorder and perhaps also in individuals with anorexia and bulimia.

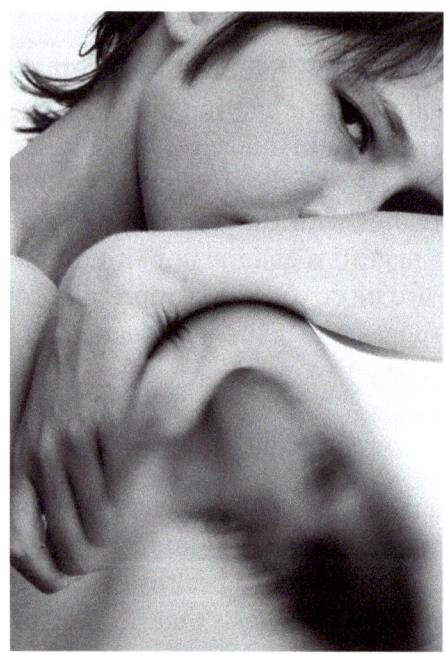

Individuals with eating disorders have been shown to develop negative affect in social situations, and therefore learn to expect others to be unavailable and insensitive to their needs.

Other

A study on the effects of priming combined event-related potential (ERP) and behavioural reactions, and investigated explicit and implicit associations between shape, weight, and self-evaluations. This was done by means of shape/weight related priming sentences and target words. ERP, reaction times, and subject ratings were collected and priming effects were analyzed. Results showed that there were stronger affective priming effects in patients with AN and BN compared to healthy controls, showing that eating disorder (ED) patients associate shape/weight concerns not only with appearance, but also nonappearance-related self-evaluation domains of interpersonal relationships and also with achievement and performance.

Social cognition is the understanding and action in interpersonal situations, and include cognitive processes involved in how people perceive and interpret information about themselves, others, and social situations. The dysfunction of social control may play a role in eating disorders. Women with ED have been shown to have lower levels of negative affect attribution compared to healthy controls, which suggests that they learn to expect others to be unavailable and insensitive to their needs. In addition, these patients were less successful at correctly encoding cause-effect relations in a social contexts and it has been suggested that their capacity to mentalize experiences is impaired. In addition to impairments in social cognition, it has been found that individuals with ED have an inability to recognize, label, and respond to different emotional states, and are impaired in visual recognition tasks.

Dementia is a disorder characterized by multiple deficits in cognition, including memory impairments. Patients with various forms of dementia have impairments in their activities of daily living including eating, and eating disorders have been found in patients with dementia. Patients with frontotemporal dementia (FTD) tend to have an eating disorder where they have food cravings and difficulty controlling the amount and type of food eaten but their memory and spatial functioning is not affected. Meanwhile patients with Alzheimer's Disease (AD), do not have this impairment, but their memory and spatial loss is negatively affected. Similar findings were shown where patients with fronto variant-frontotemporal dementia (fvFTD) show more severe and frequent symptoms of eating disorders than patients with AD. ED in patients with dementia have been tracked back to lesions in the frontal subcortical circuits including the anterior cingulate circuit, and data suggests that ED seem to be distinctive features of behavioural syndromes in groups of patients with fvFTD.

Neurobiology

Neurobiological differences have been found between individuals with eating disorders (ED) and healthy individuals. These differences are reflected in memory abilities and capabilities. Some of the main neurobiological differences are highlighted below:

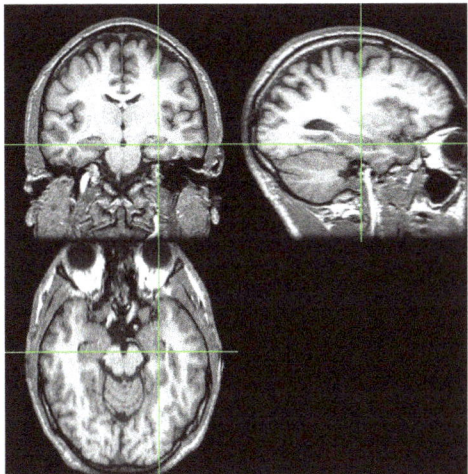

An MRI scan with the hippocampus indicated in a coronal, lateral and horizontal view.

Anorexia Nervosa

Imbalances found in certain serotonin receptor activity in cortical association regions, including the frontal lobes, are found in individuals with AN and may be the cause of impairment in their working memory, attention, motivation, and concentration. In addition, the ability of individuals with AN to activate remote memories, learn new information, plan ahead, regulate actions according to environmental stimuli, and shift behavioural sets appropriately are all implicated. Some individuals with anorexia nervosa (AN) have an inability to change their pattern response behaviours, which has been linked to disturbances found in the cortical and subgenual cingulate - mesial temporal pathways of these individuals.

The reduced blood flow in the limbic system of individuals with AN is what mostly accounts for their impairment in cognitive functioning. More specifically, the set of structures in the limbic system including the temporal lobes and adjacent structures like the hypothalamus, amygdala, and hippocampus are important in memory as well as emotion, appetite regulation, motivation, and perception, and are therefore implicated. Reduced cerebral blood flow to these areas have also been associated with impairments in complex visual memory, enhanced information processing and visuospatial ability.

Individuals with AN have been reported to have prolonged exposure to high levels of corticosteroids, a class of chemicals involved in things such as stress and behaviour, and prolonged exposure to corticosteroids has been associated with impairments in memory and learning. The hippocampus is an area of the brain that is dense with corticosteroid receptors, and therefore may be what is mediating these impairments.

Bulimia Nervosa

Activation of the medial prefrontal cortex has been shown in some studies to reflect self-schemata evaluation of relevant information, and could be used to investigate body image representations in individuals with bulimia nervosa (BN). In addition, increased activation in brain areas associated with information processing like the dorsal and anterior medial prefrontal cortex (mPFC), adjacent areas of the cingulate cortex, and the posterior cingulate and precuneus have been implicated in individuals with BN, meaning that the working memory used to actively manipulate information in these individuals is affected.

Areas of the brain such as the insula and anterior circulate cortex (ACC) have been found to be disturbed in individuals with BN. These areas are involved in self-regulation as well as executive control which controls cognitive processes including working memory, and may be the reason for impairment.

Binge Eating

An increase in dopamine in the caudate and putamen have been found in binge eaters, and studies have found a decrease in a particular serotonin transporter (5-HT) in binge eaters compared to controls. Both the caudate nucleus and putamen make up the dorsal striatum and are important as part of the brain's memory system. Dopamine is required to allow these structures to perform properly and thus this is affected in individuals with binge eating disorders, however the exact mechanism is unknown.

A dysregulation of the ventral limbic circuit has been found in individuals who binge eat. The ventral limbic circuit is important in the regulation of feeding behaviour and includes the amygdalae, insula, ventral striatum, ventral regions of the anterior ACC, and orbitofrontal cortex (OFC).

A stronger activation of the OFC has been found in patients who binge eat compared to normal weight controls, when viewing pictures of food.

Conditioning

The regulation of eating is controlled by areas of the brain involved in behaviour reinforcement. The rewarding qualities of food, including taste and smell, activate regions of the brain that are impaired in patients with anorexia nervosa (AN) and bulimia nervosa (BN), including the orbitofrontal cortex (OFC), anterior cingulate cortex (ACC), anteromedial temporal, and the insula.

Normally, eating is pleasant when an individual is hungry and less pleasant when an individual is full. Neuronal activation in the OFC decreases when an individual is full, however there is a disturbance in this pathway in individuals with AN and BN. Thus, patients with AN have little response to food or a quick response to being full, and patients with BN have an exaggerated response to food or a decrease in feeling full.

Areas of the cortex receive signals of being full by the gut through subcortical mechanisms including the thalamus which relays information from associated systems in the hypothalamus. The hypothalamus has projections into the nucleus accumbens (NAcc), which is involved in the reward system of feeding. Increased extracellular acetylcholine from interneurons in the NAcc have been found to be associated with the discontinuation of eating, and the dysregulation of this mechanism has been found in the food-reward system in eating disorder studies.

Body Image

Neurons located in different structures of the medial temporal lobe are what cause the transformation from an egocentric to an allocentric representation in space. The hippocampus generates allocentric representations for long-term memory, and the parietal cortex, retrosplenial cortex, entorhinal cortex, and hippocampus are part of a network that processes allocentric spatial information. The lateral entorhinal cortex carries nonspatial information from the perirhinal cortex to the dorsal hippocampus where it is then combined with the medial entorhinal cortex to create object-place or event-place representations in the hippocampus.

Impairment of the transformation from an egocentric to allocentric representation of oneself is what is thought to be behind the origin of obesity and eating disorders, where the egocentric perception-driven experience of an individual's real body image cannot change the allocentric memory-driven experience of a negative body, and an individual is therefore "locked" in an allocentric view of a negative representation of their body. In addition, stress and chronic stress can cause damage to the hippocampus through the overwhelming activity of the amygdala on the hippocampus.

Nutritional Deficiencies and Memory

Nutrition has proven to show effects on cognitive abilities and spatial memory. The brain's neuronal and glial cells require sufficient nutrients for energy to perform important cognitive functions such as attention and memory, and without a steady supply of nutrients including *glucose, fatty acids, and vitamins B1 (Thiamine)*, neural activation required for memory functions becomes impaired. Individuals suffering from eating disorders often lack the ability to consume the required amount of these nutrients, resulting in notable cognitive impairments such as those necessary for proper memory functioning.

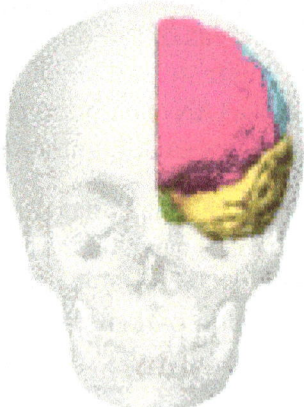

Areas of the brain effected by glucose (frontal lobe (pink), temporal lobe (yellow) and parietal lobe (blue)).

Glucose is the preferred energy source for the brain, accounting for 25% of the body's glucose consumption, despite being only 2% of the body's total weight. Glucose, along with serotonin, have been found to have significant effects within the cingulate cortex, frontal lobe, temporal lobe, and parietal lobe regions of the brain, including in those with anorexia. Individuals with eating disorders such as bulimia and anorexia show lower neural metabolism of glucose, possibly due to neural consequences of the disorder and/or due to heightened anxiety or depression. Studies have indicated the importance of glucose on memory, showing that reduced levels of glucose in the brain impair an individual's ability to retrieve memories. Most evidence suggests that severe negative impairments are due to long term, prolonged glucose deprivation or restriction, such as those seen in individuals affected by eating disorders, however effects have been studied on a more short-term basis with negative memory impairments seen in individuals who consumed breakfast compared to those who did not.

The brain contains high concentrations of lipids than any other organ in the body with the most prominent type being polyunsaturated fatty acids (PUFAs), such as omega-3 fatty acids (ω-3). Evidence that shows that low-fat intake occurs during weight loss in adolescent girls with eating disorders. Dietary ω-3 fatty acids play a particularly important role in prevention of neuropsychiatric disorders such as depression and Alzheimer's disease. Studies using animal models have expressed that ω-3 deficiencies result in diminished synaptic plasticity, impaired learning, memory and emotional coping performance later in life.

All B vitamins play a part in helping the nervous system function properly. Vitamin B1 (thiamine) is an important B vitamin and is associated with Korsakoff's syndrome, a neurological disorder due to the lack of vitamin B1. Chronic alcohol abuse is the number one cause of this syndrome, but unfortunately, even though supplementation may improve muscle co-ordination, it usually cannot reverse memory loss. Case studies have reported that the co-morbidity between eating disorders and substance abuse as a significant health issue for women, and the subgroup of patients with AN who also misuse alcohol are at particular risk of developing Korsakoff's syndrome. In other studies regarding thiamine deficiency, impairments in spatial memory, retrograde amnesia, episodic memory and working memory have all been observed.

Animal Models Used in Eating Disorders

Animal models have contributed a fair amount to the current understanding of eating disorders and obesity, in different ways and to different extents; one of the main reasons being the difference in pathophysiology of these disorders. The one specific feature of eating disorders not shared with animal behavior, is the personal choice to curtail food intake. The suitability and limitations of animal models in studies regarding human eating disorders have been discussed in various reviews. Several various types of animal models have been described which include: etiologic, isomorphic, mechanistic and predictive models.

Anorexia Nervosa

The activity-based anorexia model has been one of the most suitable animal models when studying anorexia nervosa (AN). The important behavioral aspects of AN, the drive for activity, the restricted food intake during hunger, and other physiological consequences of malnutrition, are all reproduced in this model. The "activity/stress" model produces starvation-induced immunodeficiency and various complications not observed in individuals with AN. "Separation" models involve physical separation as a stressor to induce a depression-like condition; this includes decreased feeding, weight loss, and various cognitive changes . Studies with animal models simulating loss of hunger are not well suited to replicate AN because they are essentially based on the assumption of loss of appetite.

Bulimia Nervosa

Two major factors found to contribute to binge eating in bulimia nervosa (BN) patients are: stress and negative emotions. One model of BN produces stress-induced hyperphagia, where rats go through periods of restricted food and then are allowed free access to food; this mimics the intermittent self-imposed fasting and yielding to food of BN patients. Sham-feeding rat models have been used to present the defect in the satiety mechanisms in BN due to vomiting or purging after food intake. It is known that multiple mechanisms regulate meal patterning, although in order to study them, precise consumption patterns of BN patients must be known; these intake patterns are still currently being studied.

Other models of binge eating have used various combinations of stress limited access to optional foods, and/or restriction/refeeding cycles, along with scheduled eating. These specific models have been able to address the consumptive side of BN, and have proven to be useful for testing drug effects on intake behavior. Due to the pharmacological response differences between rodents and humans, new drug development has been concentrating on drug testing specifically in human subjects.

Binge Eating Disorder

The development of animal models for binge eating has been necessary, because the mechanisms underlying the physiological and neural effects are not very well understood. Since the emotional aspects such as distress and loss of control prove difficult to model in animals, the central feature of the binge eating disorder, was attempted to be mimicked. Sham-feeding was the most prominent model used to study BED.

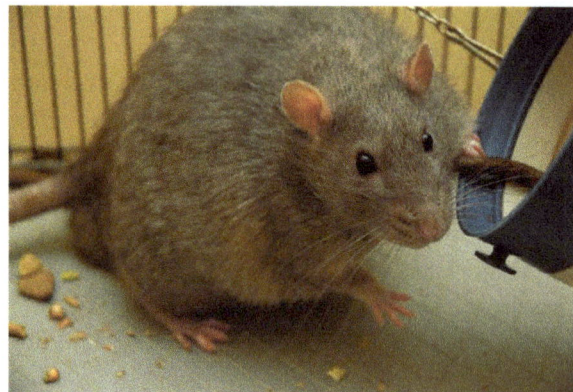

A Zucker rat which has developed diabetes due to a genetic disorder that causes obesity.

Obesity

Animal models have been able to provide key knowledge of the central and peripheral biological pathways regulating body weight and energy balance. They have proven effective and critical in examining environmental influences, along with identifying therapeutic targets and treatments. Animal models have been able to determine that malnutrition, maternal stress, and insulin injections can predispose offspring to adult obesity. Previous studies have identified the effect of the adipocyte hormone leptin, reveal that leptin treatments reverse obesity in knockout mice (ob/ob), and that diabetic (db/db) and Zucker fatty (fa/fa) rats (Zucker rat) display similar obesity phenotypes. Work on characterizing rodent obesity syndromes spontaneously arising from single gene mutations has been critical in obesity research. By 2007 there were 10 spontaneously single gene mutations characterized which deliberate an obesity phenotype. Currently, many investigators are using animal models in order to analyze genetic, neural, and physiological influences on susceptibility to diet-induced obesity.

Treatments

Neurocognitive Reserve

Cognition in individuals with anorexia nervosa (AN) has been shown to improve after treatment. It has been found that age, education, depression, body mass index (BMI), duration of illness, and length of hospitalization were not related to cognitive functioning during hospitalization and neuropsychological improvement. One of the predictors of cognitive impairment in individuals with AN is their cognitive reserve, where the greater cognitive reserve leads to more resiliency to cognitive impairment. The level of cognitive reserve predicts improvement in neuropsychological function including verbal memory, semantic fluency, basic auditory attention, and visuospatial construction. In addition, the level of cognitive reserve has been found to be associated with different AN prognosis and therefore treatment may be altered based on the cognitive reserve, where individuals who may experience more severe neurospsychological deficits may need more rehearsal and repeated practice of skills during treatment.

COMET

Low self-esteem is considered to be an important aspect of various eating disorders (ED). Implicit and opinions that refer to oneself are the main issues of low self-esteem, and competitive memory training (COMET) was developed as a treatment method for individuals with ED in order to target these opinions. COMET is aimed at making the knowledge that patients already know more easily retrieved from long-term memory by strengthening the retrieval of functional representations that are in competition with dysfunctional representations.

COMET emphasizes positive memories by using imagery, posture and facial expressions, self-verbalizations, and music. COMET stimulates emotional saliency of functional self-concepts by writing stories about scenes where positive characteristics are in action and repeatedly verbalized positive self-statements are connected to the scenes. Other techniques of COMET used to promote emotional salience include the deliberate movements of posture, facial expressions and imagery. Music that is selected by patients with ED is used to stimulate positive mood. COMET promotes higher and competitive retrieval by activating emotionally enhanced positive self-knowledge repeatedly, and then this knowledge is associated with situations and cues that trigger these dysfunctional negative self-concepts. Overall, studies have confirmed that COMET, in addition to regular therapy, enhances self-esteem in individuals with eating disorders and low self-esteem.

Virtual Reality

A reference frame is a way someone can represent their location in space, and evidence has shown that our spatial experience involves the combination of our sensory inputs from two specific reference frames including egocentric and allocentric. The ability to represent and recall objects, including our own body, changes according to our frame of references, where an egocentric stance represents objects relative to ourselves while an allocentric stance represents objects independent of ourselves. These reference frames influence how memories are stored and retrieved where in the egocentric frame, an individual sees an event from their own perspective while in the allocentric frame, an individual sees themselves engaged in the event as an observer would.

In Western culture, the body is considered a personal symbol where slenderness is associated with happiness, success and social acceptability and being overweight is associated with laziness, lack of willpower and being out of control. Social influence may therefore explain the progression from the "locked" allocentric negative body image, to obesity or eating disorders (ED) because the media and culture both promote diet and controlled eating as methods to improve body-image satisfaction. Individuals with ED are not able to use their sensory inputs to update allocentric representations of the body, therefore they hate their body even after significant weight loss and continue to attempt to improve it.

Virtual reality (VR) has been aimed at fixing this issue by helping to change the experience of the body and to improve body image in patients suffering from ED or obesity. In VR sessions, patients enter a virtual environment that causes them to face critical situations and are then helped to develop specific strategies to cope and avoid these situations. Side effects of VR include nausea and dizziness. Overall, good results were found during treatment with experiential cognitive therapy that also included specific body-image protocol based on VR in obese and binge-eating patients.

Future Research

Further research should be carried out on implicit memory and its effects and biases on eating disorders. There are conflicting results from different studies which should be resolved. Future studies can focus on correcting these implicit and explicit biases in patients with eating disorders, and see if the way these individuals affectively view and eat food can be changed by teaching these individuals how to consciously change their own thought patterns.

More research is also needed to study the specific effects of memory and attentional biases in various eating disorders. Most of the current research has been done in individuals with AN, however to gain a more comprehensive understanding of how memory impairments effect individuals with EDs, BN and EDNOS must also be looked at, and differences and similarities in memory impairments should be compared across eating disorders. Currently many animal models have provided valuable information in regard to eating disorders, but because of the cognitive and physical differences, differences do still arise. Using rodents to examine genetic etiological factors for eating disorders must patiently await breakthroughs in human studies of the same disorders.

It would be beneficial to continue research on the COMET and virtual reality treatment methods. COMET, so far, seems to be an effective intervention and the results from studies on the intervention method show that further investigation will be useful. Virtual reality is another treatment tool that has been shown to help modify locked negative body image, and good results were obtained from this study. Improvements can be made for both of these studies including better control of certain variables. The impaired memory systems have been found to be the cause of, or drive these eating disorders. If treatment methods are developed that are able to target these impaired memory systems, it could help not only to individuals in critical state but also as an intervention to individuals in the early stages to prevent their eating disorders from getting worse.

Ultimately using the present research that is available, it is important to conduct future research that expands and elaborates on what has already been discovered to find treatment options for each illness

Eating Disorders and Development

Eating disorders typically peak at specific periods in development, notably sensitive and transitional periods such as puberty. Feeding and eating disorders in childhood are often the result of a complex interplay of organic and non-organic factors. Medical conditions, developmental problems and temperament are all strongly correlated with feeding disorders, but important contextual features of the environment and parental behavior have also been found to influence the development of childhood eating disorders. Given the complexity of early childhood eating problems, consideration of both biological and behavioral factors is warranted for diagnosis and treatment.

Revisions in the DSM-5 have attempted to improve diagnostic utility for clinicians working with feeding and eating disorder patients. In the DSM-5, diagnostic categories are less defined by age of patient, and guided more by developmental differences in presentation and expression of eating problems.

Avoidant/Restrictive Intake Disorder (ARFID)

History

Avoidant/Restrictive Intake Disorder (ARFID) was added to the DSM-5 to better clinically describe a subset of eating disorder patients who previously had been diagnosed with Eating Disorder Not Otherwise Specified (EDNOS), a much broader diagnostic category with less clinical utility. Although more studies need to be conducted, initial studies are validating ARFID as a distinct eating disorder with criteria separate from Anorexia (AN) and Bulimia (BN). Patients meeting criteria for ARFID typically have a longer history of symptoms prior to diagnosis and an earlier onset than AN or BN patients. They are also more likely to have a co-morbid medical condition or anxiety disorder.

Diagnostic Criteria

An eating or feeding disturbance (e.g., apparent lack of interest in eating or food; avoidance based on sensory characteristics of food; concern about aversive consequences of eating)as manifested by persistent failure to meet appropriate nutritional and/or energy needs associated with one (or more)of the following:

1. Significant weight loss (or failure to achieve expected weight gain or faltering growth in children).

2. Significant nutritional deficiency.

3. Dependence on enteral feeding or oral nutritional supplements.

4. Marked interference with psychosocial functioning.

The disturbance is not better explained by a lack of available food or by an associated culturally sanctioned practice. The eating disturbance does not occur exclusively during the course of anorexia nervosa or bulimia nervosa, and there is no evidence of a disturbance in the way in which one's body weight or shape is experienced. The eating disturbance is not attributable to a current medical condition or not better explained by another mental disorder. When the eating disturbance occurs in the context of another condition or disorder, the severity of the eating disturbance exceeds that routinely associated with the condition or disorder and warrants additional clinical attention

Recent research suggests that patients meeting criteria for ARFID typically have a longer history of symptoms prior to diagnosis, and an earlier onset than AN or BN patients. Selective eating is persistent in ARFID patients, typically beginning in infancy or early childhood. In one recent study, they were also more likely to have a co-morbid medical condition or anxiety disorder, but less likely to have a mood disorder. At present, there is not sufficient evidence that ARFID precedes the development of a later eating disorder.

Pica

Diagnostic History

Pica is an eating disorder characterized by the ingestion of non-food or non-nutritive substances. The DSM-5 criteria for Pica are as follows:

Diagnostic Criteria

- Persistent eating of nonnutritive, nonfood substances over a period of at least 1 month.

- The eating of nonnutritive, nonfood substances is inappropriate to the developmental level of the individual.

- The eating behavior is not part of a culturally supported or socially normative practice.

- If the eating behavior occurs in the context of another mental disorder (e.g., intellectual disability [intellectual developmental disorder], autism spectrum disorder, schizophrenia) or medical condition (including pregnancy), it is sufficiently severe to warrant additional clinical attention.

For Pica to be considered, the eating of non-food items must be inappropriate to the child's developmental level, with a minimum age of two, and no upper age limit. Pica typically presents in children, but the DSM-5 specifies that it can be diagnosed at any age. Pica is most often a co-morbid condition of children with retardation or developmental disorders, but can also present as a symptom in a broader range of troubled behavior or disorders. For example, Pica is sometimes seen in individuals with schizophrenia.

Rumination Disorder

Diagnostic History

Rumination disorder (RD) is an eating disturbance characterized by the regurgitation of partially swallowed or digested food. The following are the DSM-5 criteria for RD:

- Repeated regurgitation of food over a period of at least 1 month. Regurgitated food may be re-chewed, re-swallowed, or spit out.

- The repeated regurgitation is not attributable to an associated gastrointestinal or other medical condition (e.g., gastroesophageal reflux, pyloric stenosis).

- The eating disturbance does not occur exclusively during the course of anorexia nervosa, bulimia nervosa, binge-eating disorder, or avoidant/restrictive food intake disorder.

- If the symptoms occur in the context of another mental disorder (e.g., intellectual disability [intellectual developmental disorder] or another neurodevelopmental disorder), they are sufficiently severe to warrant additional clinical attention.

Like Pica, RD most often occurs in children with mental retardation or developmental disorders. While rumination most often presents in children, the DSM-5 specifies that it can be diagnosed at any age. RD often presents slightly different in older children and adolescents in that they are less likely to re-chew the food that is brought up, and more likely to spit it out. Like Pica, rumination may also be a symptom of other disorders. For example, rumination is often a characteristic behavior of individuals with Anorexia or Bulimia. It has also been correlated with other disorders and symptoms such as anxiety and OCD.

Anorexia Nervosa

Diagnostic History

Anorexia nervosa is characterized by the severe restriction of food intake that results in a significant weight loss. There are two subtypes of Anorexia, Restricting Type and Binge-Eating/Purging Type. While historically researchers have found that Anorexia typically begins during puberty, recent epidemiological studies have found that the average age of onset of Anorexia Nervosa has moved from the previously from an average age of onset of 13-17 to a current younger age of onset of 9 -12. Among individuals with an eating disorder, 86% report the onset of the eating disorder by age 20, and 43% report the onset between the ages of 16 and 20.6. Corresponding with the age of onset, 95% of the population with current eating disorders are between the ages of 12 and 25.

Diagnostic Criteria

Anorexia is characterized by a significant reduction in energy intake which leads to a low body weight given age, sex, development, and physical health considerations.

- Individuals with anorexia also experience a significant fear of weight gain or engage in behaviors that interfere with weight gain.

- The illness is also characterized by a disturbance in body image, a significant focus and evaluation of self based on body weight, and/or lack of recognition of the consequences and seriousness of the current low body weight.

- Intense fear of gaining weight or of becoming fat, or persistent behavior that interferes with weight gain, even though at a significantly low weight.

Anorexia has two subtypes: the restricting type and the purging type. This is based on whether an individual engages in or does not engage in bingeing and purging behaviors.

Anorexia is characterized as mild, moderate, severe, or extreme based on the extent of weight loss.

Bulimia Nervosa

Bulimia nervosa is characterized by episodes of binge eating followed by inappropriate compensatory behaviors.

Diagnostic History

Similar to Anorexia, Bulimia typically begins during adolescence, though the average age of onset is somewhat later than that of anorexia. Onset before puberty and after age 40 is atypical.

Diagnostic Criteria

Bulimia is characterized by repeated episodes of binge eating following but the use of inappropriate compensatory behaviors.

- The binge eating and compensatory behaviors occur recurrently

- An individual experiences a sense of lack of control during the binge eating.

- Self evaluation is highly influenced by body image and body perceptions.

The disorder can be characterized as mild, moderate, severe, or extreme based on the number of compensatory behaviors per week. .

Binge Eating Disorder

Diagnostic History

Binge eating disorder was added as an eating disorder diagnosis in DSM-V. Previously individuals with Binge Eating Disorder had been classified under Eating Disorder Not Otherwise Specified. Due to the recency of the diagnosis, less research is currently available on Binge Eating Disorder compared to the other categories of eating disorders. The average age of onset is reported to be 25 years.

Diagnostic Criteria

Binge Eating disorder is characterized by repeated binge eating episodes. This includes:

- Eating an objectively large amount of food in a short period of time.

- Experiencing a sense of lack of control while eating.

- Feeling self-deprecating based on eating behavior.

The severity is classified by the number of binge eating episodes per week

Eating Disorder Not Otherwise Specified

Eating disorder not otherwise specified (EDNOS) is an eating disorder that does not meet the criteria for: anorexia nervosa, bulimia nervosa, or binge eating. Individuals with EDNOS usually fall into one of three groups: sub-threshold symptoms of anorexia or bulimia, mixed features of both disorders, or extremely atypical eating behaviors that are not characterized by either of the other established disorders.

People with EDNOS have similar symptoms and behaviors to those with anorexia and bulimia, and can face the same dangerous risks.

EDNOS is the most prevalent eating disorder; about 60% of adults treated for eating disorders are diagnosed with EDNOS. EDNOS occurs in both sexes.

Characteristics

Rather than providing specific diagnostic criteria for EDNOS, the fourth revision of the *Diagnostic and Statistical Manual of Mental Disorders* (*DSM-IV*) listed six non-exhaustive example presentations, including individuals who:

1. Meet all criteria for anorexia nervosa except their weight falls within the normal range

2. Meet all criteria for bulimia nervosa except they engage in binge eating or purging behaviors less than twice per week or for fewer than three months

3. Purge after eating small amounts of food while retaining a normal body weight

4. Repeatedly chew and spit out large amounts of food without swallowing

5. Do not meet criteria for binge eating disorder

Despite its subclinical status in *DSM-IV*, available data suggest that EDNOS is no less severe than the officially recognized *DSM-IV* eating disorders. In a comprehensive meta-analysis of 125 studies, individuals with EDNOS exhibited similar levels of eating pathology and general psychopathology to those with anorexia nervosa and binge eating disorder, and similar levels of physical health problems as those with anorexia nervosa. Although individuals with bulimia nervosa scored significantly higher than those with EDNOS on measures of eating pathology and general psychopathology, those with EDNOS exhibited more physical health problems than those with bulimia nervosa.

Diagnosis

The three general categories for an EDNOS diagnosis are subthreshold symptoms of anorexia or bulimia, a mixture of both anorexia or bulimia, and eating behaviors that are not particularized by anorexia and bulimia. EDNOS is no longer considered a diagnosis in *DSM-5*; those displaying symptoms of what would previously have been considered EDNOS are now classified under Other Specified Feeding or Eating Disorder.

Epidemiology

Although EDNOS (formerly called atypical eating disorder) was originally introduced in *DSM-III* to capture unusual cases, it accounts for up to 60% of cases in eating disorder specialty clinics. EDNOS is an especially prevalent category in populations that have received inadequate research attention such as young children, males, ethnic minorities, and non-Western groups.

Disordered Eating

Disordered eating describes a variety of abnormal eating behaviors that, by themselves, do not warrant diagnosis of an eating disorder.

Disordered eating includes behaviors that are common features of eating disorders, such as:

- Chronic restrained eating.
- Compulsive eating.
- Binge eating, with associated loss of control.

- Self-induced vomiting.

Disordered eating also includes behaviors that are not characteristic of any eating disorder, such as:

- Irregular, chaotic eating patterns.

- Ignoring physical feelings of hunger and satiety (fullness).

- Use of diet pills.

- Emotional eating.

- Night eating.

- "Secretive food concocting": the consumption of embarrassing food combinations, such as mashed potatoes mixed with sandwich cookies.

Potential Causes of Disordered Eating

Disordered eating can represent a change in eating patterns caused by other mental disorders (e.g. clinical depression), or by factors that are generally considered to be unrelated to mental disorders (e.g. extreme homesickness).

Certain factors among adolescents tend to be associated with disordered eating, including perceived pressure from parents and peers, nuclear family dynamic, body mass index, negative affect (mood), self-esteem, perfectionism, drug use, and participation in sports that focus on leanness. These factors are similar among boys and girls alike. However, the reported incidence rates of are consistently and significantly higher in female than male participants, with 61% of females and 28% of males reporting disordered eating behaviors in a study of over 1600 adolescents.

Nuclear Family Environment

The nuclear family dynamic of an adolescent plays a large part in the formation of their psychological, and thus behavioral, development. A research article published in the *Journal of Adolescence* concluded that, "...while families do not appear to play a primary casual role in eating pathology, dysfunctional family environments and unhealthy parenting can affect the genesis and maintenance of disordered eating."

One study explored the connection between the disordered eating patterns of adolescents and the poor socio-emotional coping mechanisms of guardians with mental disorders. It was found that in homes of parents with mental health issues (such as depression or anxiety), the children living in these environments self-reported experiencing stressful home environments, parental withdrawal, rejection, unfulfilled emotional needs, or over-involvement from their guardians. It was hypothesized that this was directly related to adolescent study participants also reporting poor emotional awareness, expression, and regulation in relation to internalized/ externalized eating disordered habits. Parental anxiety/ depression could not be directly linked to disordered eating, but could be linked to the development of poor coping skills that can lead to disordered eating behaviors.

Another study specifically investigated whether a parental's eating disorder could predict disordered eating in their children. It was found that rates of eating disorder appearances in children with either parent or the mother having a history of an eating disorder were much higher than those with parents without an eating disorder. Reported disordered eating peaked between ages 15 and 17 with the risk of eating disorder occurrences in females 12.7 times greater than of that in males. This is, "of particular interest as it has been shown that maternal ED [eating disorders] predict disordered eating behaviour in their daughters." This suggests that poor eating habits result as a coping mechanism for other direct issues presented by an unstable home environment.

Social Stresses

Additional stress from outside the home environment influence disordered eating characteristics. Social stresses from peer environments, such as feeling out of place or discriminated against, has been shown to increase feelings of body shame and social anxiety in studies of minority groups that lead to a prevalence of disordered eating.

A study published in the *International Journal of Eating Disorders* used data from the Massachusetts Youth Risk Behavior Surveys from 1999 to 2013 to examine how disordered eating has trended in heterosexual versus LGB (lesbian, gay, bisexual) youth. The data from over 26,000 surveys investigated the practices of purging, fasting, and using diet pills. It was found that, "sexual minority youth report disproportionately higher prevalence of disordered eating compared to heterosexual peers: up to 1 in 4 sexual minority youth report...patterns of disordered eating..." In addition, the gap between the number of LGBT females and heterosexual females controlling weight in unhealthy ways has continued to widen.

The concept this study proposed to explain this disparity comes from the minority stress theory. This states that unhealthy behaviors are directly related to the distal stress, or social stress, that minorities experience. These stressors could include rejection or pressure by peers, and physical, mental, and/ or emotional harassment.

A study published in *Psychology of Women Quarterly* explored the connection between social anxiety stresses and eating disordered habits more in depth in women in the LGBTQ community who were also racial minorities. Over 450 women ranked their interactions with every-day discrimination, their LGBTQ identity, social anxiety, their objectified body consciousness, and an eating disorder inventory diagnostic scale. The findings of the compilation of survey responses indicated that increased discrimination led to proximal minority stress, leading to feelings of social anxiety and body shame, which could be directly associated with binge eating, bulimia, and other signs of disordered eating. It has also been suggested that being a "double" or "triple" minority who experiences discrimination towards multiple characteristics contributes to more intense psychological distress and maladaptive coping mechanisms.

Athletic Influences

Disordered eating among athletes, particularly female athletes, has been the subject of much research. In one study, women with disordered eating were 3.6 times as likely to have an eating disorder if they were athletes. In addition, female collegiate athletes who compete in heavily body conscious sports like gymnastics, swimming, or diving are shown to be more at risk for developing an eating disorder. This is a result of the engagement in sports where weekly repeated weigh-ins are standard, and usually required by coaches.

A study published in *Eating Behaviors* examined the pressure of mandated weigh-ins on female collegiate athletes and how that pressure was dealt with in terms of weight management. After analyzing over 400 survey responses, it was found that athletes reported increased uses of diet pills/laxatives, consuming less calories than needed for their sport, and following nutrition information from unqualified sources. 75% of the weighed athletes reported using a weight-management method such as restricting food intake, increasing exercise, eating low fat foods, taking laxatives, vomiting, and other.

These habits were found to be worse in athletes that were weighed in front of their peers than those weighed in private. In addition, especially in gymnasts, preoccupation and anxiety about gaining weight and being weighed, and viewing food as the enemy were prevalent mindsets. This harmful mindset continued even after the gymnasts were retired from their sport: "Although retired, these gymnasts were still afraid to step onto a scale, were anxious about gaining weight…suggesting that the negative effects of being weighed can linger…[and] suggest[ing] that the weight/ fitness requirements acted as a socio-cultural pressure that would substantially increase the women's risk of developing an disordered eating in the future."

Disordered eating, along with amenorrhea and bone demineralization, form what clinicians refer to as the female athletic triad, or FAT. In contribution to these eating disorders that these female athletes develop, Results in the lack of nutrition. This can lead to the loss of several or more consecutive periods which then leads to calcium and bone loss, putting the athlete at great risk of fracturing bones and damaging tissues. Each of these conditions is a medical concern as they create serious health risks that may be life threatening to the individual. While any female athlete can develop the triad, adolescent girls are considered most at risk because of the active biological changes and growth spurts that they experience, rapidly changing life circumstances that are observed within the teenage years, and peer and social pressures.

Social Media

Researchers have said the most pervasive and influential factor controlling body image perception is the mass media. One study examined the impact of celebrity and peer Instagram images on women's body image as, "comparisons will be most readily made with individuals who are perceived as being similar" to the target as there is more of a relationship between the two parties. The participants in this study,138 female undergraduate students ages 18–30, were shown 15 images each of attractive celebrities, attractive unknown peers, and travel destinations. The participant's reactions were observed and visual scales were used to measure mood and dissatisfaction before and after viewing the images. The findings of this experiment determined that negative mood and body dissatisfaction rankings were greater after being exposed to the celebrity and peer images, with no difference between celebrity versus peer images. The media is especially dangerous for females at risk for developing body image issues, and disordered eating, because the sheer number of possible comparisons become larger.

Binge Eating

Binge eating is a pattern of disordered eating which consists of episodes of uncontrollable eating. It is sometimes a symptom of binge eating disorder or compulsive overeating disorder. During such binges, a person rapidly consumes an excessive quantity of food. A diagnosis of binge eating is associated with feelings of loss of control.

Behaviour

Typically the eating is done rapidly and a person will feel emotionally numb and unable to stop eating. Most people who have eating binges try to hide this behavior from others, and often feel ashamed about being overweight or depressed about their overeating. Although people who do not have any eating disorder may occasionally experience episodes of overeating, frequent binge eating is often a symptom of an eating disorder.

Binge-eating disorder, as the name implies, is characterized by uncontrollable, excessive eating, followed by feelings of shame and guilt. Unlike those with bulimia, those with binge-eating disorder symptoms typically do not purge their food, fast, or excessively exercise to compensate for binges. Additionally, these individuals tend to diet more often, enroll in weight-control programs and have a history of family obesity. However, many who have bulimia also have binge-eating disorder.

Emotional Eating

Emotional eating is defined as overeating in order to relieve negative emotions. Thus, emotional eating is considered a maladaptive coping strategy. If an individual frequently engages in emotional eating, it can increase the risk of developing other eating disorders, like bulimia and anorexia nervosa. Research has also shown that the presence of an existing eating disorder increases the likelihood that an individual will engage in emotional eating. Given the relationship between serious eating disorders and emotional eating behavior, it is important for clinical psychologists and nutritionists to recognize the signs of emotional eating and provide individuals with treatment. Since emotional eating is utilized to manage negative emotions, treatment necessitates learning healthy and more effective coping strategies.

Background

Emotional eating is a form of disordered eating and is defined as "an increase in food intake in response to negative emotions" and can be considered a maladaptive strategy used to cope with difficult feelings. More specifically, emotional eating would qualify as a form of emotion-focused coping, which attempts to minimize, regulate and prevent emotional distress. Interestingly, a study conducted by Bennett et al. found that emotional eating sometimes does not reduce emotional distress but instead enhances emotional distress by sparking feelings of intense guilt after an emotional eating session. Not only is emotional eating a poor way to cope, but those individuals who frequently utilize emotional eating to cope with social or psychological stressors are at an increased risk of developing eating disorders. Emotional eaters are at an especially high risk of developing binge-eating disorder. 2.8% of Americans struggle with binge-eating disorder, which increases their risk of developing cardiovascular disease and high blood pressure. At the same time, the presence of other eating disorders increases the risk of an individual engaging in emotional eating. In a clinical setting, emotional eating disorders can be diagnosed by the Dutch Eating Behavior Questionnaire which contains a scale for restrained, emotional and external eating. While therapists may use positive psychology as a way to reduce the negative emotions that trigger emotional eating, reappraisal is often a complementary treatment with the primary treatment being focused on developing alternative coping strategies.

Major Theories

Current research suggests that certain individual factors may increase one's likelihood of using emotional eating as a coping strategy. The inadequate affect regulation theory posits that individuals engage in emotional eating because they believe overeating alleviates negative feelings. Escape theory builds upon inadequate affect regulation theory by suggesting that people not only overeat to cope with negative emotions, but they find that overeating diverts their attention away from a stimuli that is threatening self-esteem to focus on a pleasurable stimuli like food. Restraint theory suggests that overeating as a result of negative emotions occurs among individuals who already restrain their eating. While these individuals typically limit what they eat, when they are faced with negative emotions they cope by engaging in emotional eating. Restraint theory supports the idea that individuals with other eating disorders are more likely to engage in emotional eating. Together these three theories suggest that an individual's aversion to negative emotions, particularly negative feelings that arise in response to a threat to the ego or intense self-awareness, increase the propensity for the individual to utilize emotional eating as a means of coping with this aversion.

The biological stress response may also contribute to the development of emotional eating tendencies. In a crisis, corticotropin-releasing hormone (CRH) is secreted by the hypothalamus, suppressing appetite and triggering the release of glucocorticoids from the adrenal gland. These steroid hormones increase appetite and, unlike CRH, remain in the bloodstream for a prolonged period of time, often resulting in hyperphagia. Those who experience this biologically instigated increase in appetite during times of stress are therefore primed to rely on emotional eating as a coping mechanism.

Contributing Factors

Negative Affect

Overall, high levels of the negative affect trait are related to emotional eating. Negative affectivity is a personality trait involving negative emotions and poor self-concept. It has been found that certain negative affect regulation scales predicted emotional eating. Additionally, a study conducted by Bennett et al. found that individuals engage in emotional eating only when they are experiencing negative emotions. More specifically, an inability to articulate and identify one's emotions made the individual feel inadequate at regulating negative affect and thus more likely to engage in emotional eating. A study conducted by Spoor et al. attempted to further delineate the relationship between negative affect and emotional eating. They found that negative affect was not significantly related to emotional eating when taking into consideration emotion focused coping and avoidance distraction behavior. This suggests that negative affect is not independently related to emotional eating but is instead indirectly related through emotional focused coping and avoidance distraction behavior. While Spence and Spoor's findings differed somewhat, they both suggest that negative affect does play a role in emotional eating but it may be accounted for by other variables.

Related disorders

Emotional eating itself may be a precursor to developing eating disorders such as binge eating or bulimia nervosa. The relationship between emotional eating and other disorders is largely due to the fact that that emotional eating and these disorders share key characteristics. More specifically, they are both related to emotion focused coping, maladaptive coping strategies, and a strong aversion to negative feelings and stimuli. It is important to note that the causal direction has not been definitively established, meaning that while emotional eating is considered a precursor to these eating disorders, it may be also be the consequence of these disorders. The latter hypothesis that emotional eating happens in response to another eating disorder is supported by research that has shown emotional eating to be more common among individuals already suffering from bulimia nervosa.

Biological and Environmental Factors

Individual differences in the physiological stress response may also contribute to the development of emotional eating habits. Those whose adrenal glands naturally secrete larger quantities of glucocorticoids in response to a stressor are more inclined toward hyperphagia, which can act as a physiological catalyst for emotional eating. Additionally, those whose bodies require more time to clear the bloodstream of excess glucocorticoids are similarly predisposed. These biological factors can interact with environmental elements to further trigger hyperphagia, namely the type of stressor the individual is subjected to. Frequent intermittent stressors trigger repeated, sporadic releases of glucocorticoids broken up by intervals too short to allow for a complete return to baseline levels, leading to increased appetite. Those whose lifestyles or careers entail frequent intermittent stressors thus have greater biological incentive to develop patterns of emotional eating.

Impact

Emotional eating may qualify as avoidant coping and/or emotion-focused coping. As coping methods that fall under these broad categories focus on temporary reprieve rather than practical resolution of stressors, they can initiate a vicious cycle of maladaptive behavior reinforced by fleeting relief from stress. Additionally, in the presence of high insulin levels characteristic of the recovery phase of the stress-response, glucocorticoids trigger the creation of an enzyme that stores away the nutrients circulating in the bloodstream after an episode of emotional eating as visceral fat, or fat located in the abdominal area. Therefore, those who struggle with emotional eating are at greater risk for abdominal obesity, which is in turn linked to a greater risk for metabolic and cardiovascular disease.

Treatment

There are numerous ways in which individuals can reduce emotional distress without engaging in emotional eating. The most salient choice is to minimize maladaptive coping strategies and to maximize adaptive strategies. A study conducted by Corstorphine et al. in 2007 investigated the relationship between distress tolerance and disordered eating. These researchers specifically focused on how different coping strategies impact distress tolerance and disordered eating. They found that individuals who engage in disordered eating often employ emotional avoidance strategies. If an individual is faced with strong negative emotions, they may choose to avoid the situation by distracting themselves through overeating. Discouraging emotional avoidance is thus an important facet to emotional eating treatment. The most obvious way to limit emotional avoidance is to confront the issue through techniques like problem solving. Corstorphine et al. showed that individuals who engaged in problem solving strategies enhance one's ability to tolerate emotional distress. Since emotional distress is correlated to emotional eating, the ability to better manage one's negative affect should allow an individual to cope with a situation without resorting to overeating.

One way to combat emotional eating is to employ mindfulness techniques. For example, approaching cravings with a nonjudgmental inquisitiveness can help differentiate between hunger and emotionally-driven cravings. An individual may ask his or herself if the craving developed rapidly, as emotional eating tends to be triggered spontaneously. An individual may also take the time to note his or her bodily sensations, such as hunger pangs, and coinciding emotions, like guilt or shame, in order to make conscious decisions to avoid emotional eating.

Emotional eating disorder predisposes individuals to more serious eating disorders and physiological complications. Therefore, combatting disordered eating before such progression takes place has become the focus of many clinical psychologists.

Ingestive Behaviors

Ingestive behaviors encompass all eating and drinking behaviors. These actions are influenced by physiological regulatory mechanisms; these mechanisms exist to control and establish homeostasis within the human body. Disruptions in these ingestive regulatory mechanisms can result in eating disorders such as obesity, anorexia, and bulimia.

Research has confirmed that physiological mechanisms play an important role in homeostasis; however, human food intake must also be evaluated within the context of non-physiological determinants present in human life. Within laboratory environments, hunger and satiety are factors that can be controlled and tested. Outside of experiments though, social constraints may influence the size and number of daily meals.

Initiating Ingestion

Body weight regulation requires a balance between food intake and energy expenditure. Two mechanisms are required to maintain a relatively constant body weight: one must increase motivation to eat if long-term reservoirs are being depleted, and the other must restrain food intake if more calories than needed are being consumed.

Signals from Environment

The environment of early humans shaped the evolution of ingestive regulatory mechanisms, starvation used to be a greater threat to survival than overeating. Human metabolism evolved to store energy within the body to prevent death from starvation. Today, the environment now has an opposite effect on humans eating behaviors. With the widespread availability of food in today's society, concern has shifted from starvation to overeating. As food scarcity and availability have become less and less of a problem, food intake has increased. The increase of food intake by so many people is due primarily to a number of environmental factors. Main social environmental factors include:

- People who eat in groups tend to eat more than when they are by themselves

- When people eat in the presence of models who eat a lot or a little, they are likely to eat similarly to the model

- Individuals who eat in the presence of others who they think are watching them, tend to eat less than they do when they are by themselves

- Along with social environmental factors, ingestive behaviors are also influenced by atmospheric environmental factors. Atmospheric factors include:

- Package Sizing: the size of the packaging tends to influence what an individual thinks is the norm for cosumption

- Food Odor: unpleasant odors are likely to decrease ingestion, while pleasant odors are likely to increase ingestion

- Temperature of environment: people tend to eat more in cold climates and tend to drink more in warmer climates

- Lighting of Environment: people are more likely to stay put and eat in an environment with dim lighting rather than harsh bright lighting

Signals from Stomach

The gastrointestinal system, particularly the stomach, releases a peptide hormone called ghrelin. In 1999 experiments have revealed that hunger is communicated from the stomach to the brain via this hormone peptide. This peptide can stimulate thought about food, and is suppressed after food is ingested. Nutrient injection into the blood stream does not suppress ghrelin, so the release of hormone is directed by the digestive system and not by nutrient availability in the blood. These blood levels of ghrelin increase with fasting and are reduced after a meal. Ghrelin antibodies or ghrelin receptor antagonists inhibit eating. Ghrelin also stimulates energy production and signals directly to the hypothalamus regulatory nucli that control energy homeostasis.

Metabolic Signals

Hunger is the result of a fall in blood glucose level or depriving cells of the ability to metabolize fatty acids - glucoprivation and lipoprivation, respectively, stimulate eating. Detectors in the brain are only sensitive to glucoprivation; detectors in the liver are sensitive to both glucoprivation and lipoprivation outside the blood–brain barrier. However, no single set of receptors is solely responsible for the information the brain uses to control eating.

Satiety signals

There are two primary sources of signals that stop eating: short-term signals come from immediate effects of eating a meal, beginning before food digestion, and long-term signals, that arise in adipose tissue, control the intake of calories by monitoring the sensitivity of brain mechanisms to hunger and satiety signals received.

Short-term Signals

Head Factors

There are several sets of receptors located in the head: eyes, nose, tongue, and throat. The most important role of head factors in satiety is that taste and odor can serve as stimuli that permit learning about caloric contents of different foods. Tasting and swallowing of food contributes to the feeling of fullness caused by the presence of food in the stomach.

Gastric and Intestinal Factors

The stomach contains receptors that can detect the presence of nutrients, but there are detectors in the intestines as well, and the satiety factors of the stomach and intestines can interact. Cholecystokinin (CCK) is a peptide hormone secreted by the duodenum that controls the rate of stomach emptying. CCK is secreted in response to the presence of fats, which are detected in by receptors in the duodenum. Another satiety signal produced by cells is peptide YY_{3-36} (PYY), which is released after a meal in amounts proportional to the calories ingested.

Liver Factors

The last stage of satiety occurs in the liver. The liver is also the first organ to detect that nutrients are being received from the intestines. When the liver receives nutrients, it then sends a signal to the brain that produces satiety; but essentially, it is continuing the satiety that was already started by signals that arose from the stomach and upper intestine.

Long-term Signals

Signals arising from the long-term nutrient reservoir of the body may alter the sensitivity of the brain to hunger signals or short-term satiety signals. A peptide, leptin, has profound effects on metabolism and eating. It is secreted by adipose tissue and it increases metabolic rate while decreasing food intake. Its discovery has stimulated interest in finding ways of treating obesity.

Brain Mechanisms

Neural circuits in the brain stem are able to control acceptance or rejection of sweet or bitter foods, and can be modulated by satiation or physiological hunger signals. Signals from the tongue, stomach, small intestine and liver are received by the area postrema and nucleus of the solitary tract, which then send information to many regions of the forebrain that control food intake. The lateral hypothalamus contains two sets of neurons that increase eating and decrease metabolic rate by secreting the peptides orexin and melanin concentrating hormone (MCH). Neuropeptide Y (NPY) in the lateral hypothalamus induces ravenous eating; neurons that secrete NPY are targeted by ghrelin in the hypothalamus. Leptin desensitizes the brain to hunger signals and inhibits NPY-secreting neurons.

References

- Shafran, R., Lee, M., Cooper, Z., Palmer, R. L., & Fairburn, C. G. (2007). Attentional bias in eating disorders. The International Journal of Eating Disorders (Print), 40(4), 369-380

- Butow, P. Beaumont, P. & Touyz, S. (1993) Cognitive processes in dieting disorders. International Journal of Eating Disorders, 14, 319-329

- Teckcan, A. İ., Taş, A. Ç., Topçuoğlu, V., & Yücel, B. (2008). Memory bias in anorexia nervosa: Evidence from directed forgetting. Journal of Behavior Therapy and Experimental Psychiatry, 39(3), 369-380

- American Psychiatric Association. Diagnostic and Statistical Manual of Mental Disorders. 4th, text revision (DSM-IV-TR) ed. 2000. ISBN 0-89042-334-2. Dementia

- King, G. A., Polivy, J., & Herman, C. P. (1991). Cognitive aspects of dietary restraint: Effects on person memory. International Journal of Eating Disorders, 10, 313–321

- Legenbauer, T., Maul, B., Rühl, I., Kleinstäuber, M., & Hiller, W. (2010). Memory bias for schema-related stimuli in individuals with bulimia nervosa. Journal of Clinical Psychology, 66(3), 302-316

- Hermans, D., Pieters, G., Eelen, P. (1998). Implicit and explicit memory for shape, body weight and food-related words in patients with anorexia nervosa and nondieting controls. Journal of Abnormal Psychology. 193–202

- American Psychiatric Association (2013). The Diagnostic and Statistical Manual of Mental Disorders. American Psychiatric Association. pp. 329–354. ISBN 9780890425541

- Newcomer, J.W., Craft, S., Hershey, T., Askins, K., & Bardgett, M.E. (1994). Glucocorticoid-induced impairment in declarative memory in adult humans. Journal of Neuroscience 14, 2047–2053

- Wolkowitz, O.M., Reus, V.I., Weingartner, H., Thompson, K., Brier, A., Doran, A., Rubinow, D., & Pickar, D. (1990). Cognitive effects of corticosteroids. American Journal of Psychiatry 147, 1297–1303

- Riva, G. (2011) The key to unlocking the virtual body: Virtual Reality in the Treatment of Obesity and Eating Disorders. Journal of Diabetes Science and Technology. 2, 5, 283 – 292

- Delvenne, V., Goldman, S., & Lotstra, F. (1999). Brain glucose metabolism in eatingdisorders assessed by positron emission tomography. International Journal of Eating Disorders, 25(1), 29-37

- Bryant-Waugh, Rachel; Laura Markham; Richard Kreipe; Timothy Walsh (8 Jan 2010). "Feeding and Eating Disorders in Childhood". International Journal of Eating Disorders. 43 (2): 98–111. doi:10.1002/eat.20795

- Fisher, Martin (19 Nov 2013). "Characteristics of Avoidant/Restrictive Food Intake Disorder in Children and Adolescents". Journal of Adolescent Health. doi:10.1016/j.jadohealth.2013.11.013. Retrieved 15 Apr 2014

2

Types of Eating Disorders

Eating disorders can be of various types like anorexia nervosa, bulimia nervosa, binge eating disorder and muscle dysmorphia. Anorexia nervosa is a psychological disorder which is defined by an extremely low body weight whereas binge eating disorder leads to uncontrollable eating. The major categories of eating disorders are dealt with great details in the chapter.

Anorexia Nervosa

Anorexia nervosa, often referred to simply as anorexia, is an eating disorder characterized by a low weight, fear of gaining weight, a strong desire to be thin, and food restriction. Many people with anorexia see themselves as overweight even though they are in fact underweight. If asked they usually deny they have a problem with low weight. Often they weigh themselves frequently, eat only small amounts, and only eat certain foods. Some will exercise excessively, force themselves to vomit, or use laxatives to produce weight loss. Complications may include osteoporosis, infertility and heart damage, among others. Women will often stop having menstrual periods.

The cause is not known. There appear to be some genetic components with identical twins more often affected than non-identical twins. Cultural factors also appear to play a role with societies that value thinness having higher rates of disease. Additionally, it occurs more commonly among those involved in activities that value thinness such as high-level athletics, modelling, and dancing. Anorexia often begins following a major life-change or stress-inducing event. The diagnosis requires a significantly low weight. The severity of disease is based on body mass index (BMI) in adults with mild disease having a BMI of greater than 17, moderate a BMI of 16 to 17, severe a BMI of 15 to 16, and extreme a BMI less than 15. In children a BMI for age percentile of less than the 5th percentile is often used.

Treatment of anorexia involves restoring a healthy weight, treating the underlying psychological problems, and addressing behaviors that promote the problem. While medications do not help with weight gain, they may be used to help with associated anxiety or depression. A number of types of therapy may be useful including an approach where parents assume responsibility for feeding their child, known as Maudsley family therapy and cognitive behavioral therapy. Sometimes people require admission to hospital to restore weight. Evidence for benefit from nasogastric tube feeding, however, is unclear. Some people will just have a single episode and recover while others may have many episodes over years. Many complications improve or resolve with regaining of weight.

Globally, anorexia is estimated to affect 2.9 million people as of 2015. It is estimated to occur in 0.9% to 4.3% of women and 0.2% to 0.3% of men in Western countries at some point in their life. About 0.4% of young females are affected in a given year and it is estimated to occur ten times less commonly in males. Rates in most of the developing world are unclear. Often it begins during the teen years or young adulthood. While anorexia became more commonly diagnosed during the 20th century it is unclear if this was due to an increase in its frequency or simply better diagnosis. In 2013 it directly resulted in about 600 deaths globally, up from 400 deaths in 1990. Eating disorders also increase a person's risk of death from a wide range of other causes, including suicide. About 5% of people with anorexia die from complications over a ten-year period, a nearly 6 times increased risk. The term anorexia nervosa was first used in 1873 by William Gull to describe this condition.

Signs and Symptoms

Anorexia nervosa is an eating disorder characterized by attempts to lose weight, to the point of starvation. A person with anorexia nervosa may exhibit a number of signs and symptoms, the type and severity of which may vary and may be present but not readily apparent.

Anorexia nervosa, and the associated malnutrition that results from self-imposed starvation, can cause complications in every major organ system in the body. Hypokalaemia, a drop in the level of potassium in the blood, is a sign of anorexia nervosa. A significant drop in potassium can cause abnormal heart rhythms, constipation, fatigue, muscle damage and paralysis.

Symptoms may include:

- A low body mass index for one's age and height.

- Amenorrhea, a symptom that occurs after prolonged weight loss; causes menses to stop, hair becomes brittle, and skin becomes yellow and unhealthy.

- Fear of even the slightest weight gain; taking all precautionary measures to avoid weight gain or becoming "overweight".

- Rapid, continuous weight loss.

- Lanugo: soft, fine hair growing over the face and body.

- An obsession with counting calories and monitoring fat contents of food.

- Preoccupation with food, recipes, or cooking; may cook elaborate dinners for others, but not eat the food themselves or consume a very small portion.

- Food restrictions despite being underweight or at a healthy weight.

- Food rituals, such as cutting food into tiny pieces, refusing to eat around others and hiding or discarding of food.

- Purging: May use laxatives, diet pills, ipecac syrup, or water pills to flush food out of their system after eating or may engage in self-induced vomiting though this is a more common symptom of bulimia.

- Excessive exercise including micro-exercising, for example making small persistent movements of fingers or toes.

- Perception of self as overweight, in contradiction to an underweight reality.

- Intolerance to cold and frequent complaints of being cold; body temperature may lower (hypothermia) in an effort to conserve energy due to malnutrition.

- Hypotension or orthostatic hypotension.

- Bradycardia or tachycardia.

- Depression, anxiety disorders and insomnia.

- Solitude: may avoid friends and family and become more withdrawn and secretive.

- Abdominal distension.

- Halitosis (from vomiting or starvation-induced ketosis).

- Dry hair and skin, as well as hair thinning.

- Chronic fatigue.

- Rapid mood swings.

- Having feet discoloration causing an orange appearance.

- Having severe muscle tension + aches and pains.

- Evidence/habits of self harming or self-loathing.

- Admiration of thinner people.

Associated Problems

Other psychological issues may factor into anorexia nervosa; some fulfill the criteria for a separate Axis I diagnosis or a personality disorder which is coded Axis II and thus are considered comorbid to the diagnosed eating disorder. Some people have a previous disorder which may increase their vulnerability to developing an eating disorder and some develop them afterwards. The presence of Axis I or Axis II psychiatric comorbidity has been shown to affect the severity and type of anorexia nervosa symptoms in both adolescents and adults.

Obsessive-compulsive disorder (OCD) and obsessive-compulsive personality disorder (OCPD) are highly comorbid with AN, particularly the restrictive subtype. Obsessive-compulsive personality disorder is linked with more severe symptomatology and worse prognosis. The causality between personality disorders and eating disorders has yet to be fully established. Other comorbid conditions include depression, alcoholism, borderline and other personality disorders, anxiety disorders, attention deficit hyperactivity disorder, and body dysmorphic disorder (BDD). Depression and anxiety are the most common comorbidities, and depression is associated with a worse outcome.

Autism spectrum disorders occur more commonly among people with eating disorders than in the general population. Zucker *et al.* (2007) proposed that conditions on the autism spectrum make up the cognitive endophenotype underlying anorexia nervosa and appealed for increased interdisciplinary collaboration.

Causes

There is evidence for biological, psychological, developmental, and sociocultural risk factors, but the exact cause of eating disorders is unknown.

Biological

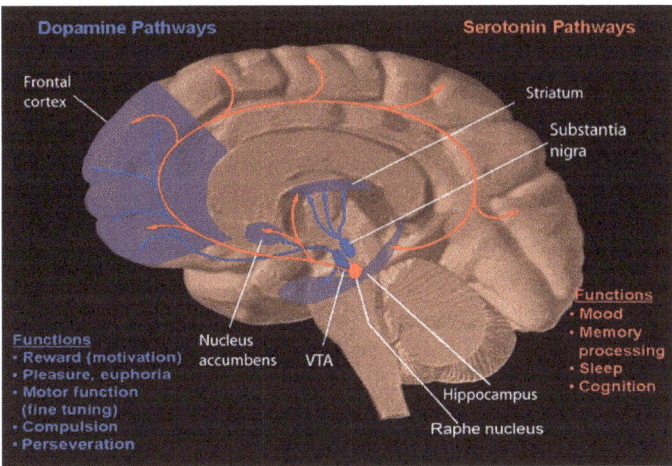

Dysregulation of the serotonin pathways has been implicated in the etiology, pathogenesis and pathophysiology of anorexia nervosa.

- Genetics: anorexia nervosa is highly heritable. Twin studies have shown a heritability rate of between 28 and 58%. Association studies have been performed, studying 128 different polymorphisms related to 43 genes including genes involved in regulation of eating behavior, motivation and reward mechanics, personality traits and emotion. Consistent associations have been identified for polymorphisms associated with agouti-related peptide, brain derived neurotrophic factor, catechol-o-methyl transferase, SK3 and opioid receptor delta-1. Epigenetic modifications, such as DNA methylation, may contribute to the development or maintenance of anorexia nervosa, though clinical research in this area is in its infancy.

- Obstetric complications: prenatal and perinatal complications may factor into the development of anorexia nervosa, such as maternal anemia, diabetes mellitus, preeclampsia, placental infarction, and neonatal cardiac abnormalities. Neonatal complications may also have an influence on harm avoidance, one of the personality traits associated with the development of AN.

- Neuroendocrine dysregulation: altered signalling of peptides that facilitate communication between the gut, brain and adipose tissue, such as ghrelin, leptin, neuropeptide Y and orexin, may contribute to the pathogenesis of anorexia nervosa by disrupting regulation of hunger and satiety.

- Gastrointestinal diseases: people with gastrointestinal disorders may be more risk of developing disorders eating practices than the general population, principally restrictive eating disturbances. An association of anorexia nervosa with celiac disease has been found. The role that gastrointestinal symptoms play in the development of eating disorders seems rather complex. Some authors report that unresolved symptoms prior to gastrointestinal disease diagnosis may create a food aversion in these persons, causing alterations to their eating patterns. Other authors report that greater symptoms throughout their diagnosis led to greater risk. It has been documented that some people with celiac disease, irritable bowel syndrome or inflammatory bowel disease who are not conscious about the importance of strictly following their diet, choose to consume their trigger foods to promote weight loss. On the other hand, individuals with good dietary management may develop anxiety, food aversion and eating disorders because of concerns around cross contamination of their foods. Some authors suggest that medical professionals should evaluate the presence of an unrecognized celiac disease in all people with eating disorder, especially if they present any gastrointestinal symptom (such as decreased appetite, abdominal pain, bloating, distension, vomiting, diarrhea or constipation), weight loss, or growth failure; and also routinely ask celiac patients about weight or body shape concerns, dieting or vomiting for weight control, to evaluate the possible presence of eating disorders, specially in women.

Studies have hypothesized the continuance of disordered eating patterns may be epiphenomena of starvation. The results of the Minnesota Starvation Experiment showed normal controls exhibit many of the behavioral patterns of anorexia nervosa (AN) when subjected to starvation. This may be due to the numerous changes in the neuroendocrine system, which results in a self-perpetuating cycle.

Another hypothesis is that anorexia nervosa is more likely to occur in populations in which obesity is more prevalent, and results from a sexually selected evolutionary drive to appear youthful in populations in which size becomes the primary indicator of age.

Anorexia nervosa is more likely to occur in a person's pubertal years. Some explanatory hypotheses for the rising prevalence of eating disorders in adolescence are "increase of adipose tissue in girls, hormonal changes of puberty, societal expectations of increased independence and autonomy that are particularly difficult for anorexic adolescents to meet; [and] increased influence of the peer group and its values."

Psychological

Early theories of the cause of anorexia linked it to childhood sexual abuse or dysfunctional families; evidence is conflicting, and well-designed research is needed. The fear of food is known as *sitiophobia*, *cibophobia*, or *sitophobia* and is part of the differential diagnosis. Other psychological causes of anorexia include low self-esteem, feeling like there is lack of control, depression, anxiety, and loneliness.

Sociological

Anorexia nervosa has been increasingly diagnosed since 1950; the increase has been linked to vulnerability and internalization of body ideals. People in professions where there is a particular social pressure to be thin (such as models and dancers) were more likely to develop anorexia, and those with anorexia have much higher contact with cultural sources that promote weight loss. This trend can also be observed for people who partake in certain sports, such as jockeys and wrestlers. There is a higher incidence and prevalence of anorexia nervosa in sports with an emphasis on aesthetics, where low body fat is advantageous, and sports in which one has to make weight for competition. Family dynamics can play big part in the cause of anorexia. When there is a constant pressure from people to be thin, teasing, bullying can cause low self-esteem and other psychological symptoms.

Media Effects

Constant exposure to media that presents body ideals may constitute a risk factor for body dissatisfaction and anorexia nervosa. The cultural ideal for body shape for men versus women continues to favor slender women and athletic, V-shaped muscular men. A 2002 review found that, of the magazines most popular among people aged 18 to 24 years, those read by men, unlike those read by women, were more likely to feature ads and articles on shape than on diet. Body dissatisfaction and internalization of body ideals are risk factors for anorexia nervosa that threaten the health of both male and female populations.

Websites that stress the importance of attainment of body ideals extol and promote anorexia nervosa through the use of religious metaphors, lifestyle descriptions, "thinspiration" or "fitspiration" (inspirational photo galleries and quotes that aim to serve as motivators for attainment of body ideals). Pro-anorexia websites reinforce internalization of body ideals and the importance of their attainment.

The media give men and women a false view of what people truly look like. In magazines, movies and even on billboards most of the actors/models are photoshopped in multiple ways. People then strive to look like these "perfect" role models when in reality they aren't any where near perfection themselves.

Mechanisms

- Serotonin dysregulation: brain imaging studies implicate alterations of 5-HT1A and 5-HT2A receptors and the 5-HT transporter. Alterations of these circuits may affect mood and impulse control as well as the motivating and hedonic aspects of feeding behavior. Starvation has been hypothesized to be a response to these effects, as it is known to lower tryptophan and steroid hormone metabolism, which might reduce serotonin levels at these critical sites and ward off anxiety.

- Addiction to the chemicals released in the brain during starving and physical activity: people affected with anorexia often report getting some sort of high from not eating. The effect of food restriction and intense activity causes symptoms similar to anorexia in female rats, though it is not explained why this addiction affects only females.

- Resting state fMRI has identified the insular cortex and corticolimbic circuitry as likely brain areas responsible for the symptomology of anorexia nervosa.

Diagnosis

A diagnostic assessment includes the person's current circumstances, biographical history, current symptoms, and family history. The assessment also includes a mental state examination, which is an assessment of the person's current mood and thought content, focusing on views on weight and patterns of eating.

DSM-5

Anorexia nervosa is classified under the Feeding and Eating Disorders in the latest revision of the *Diagnostic and Statistical Manual of Mental Disorders* (DSM 5).

Relative to the previous version of the DSM (DSM-IV-TR), the 2013 revision (DSM5) reflects changes in the criteria for anorexia nervosa, most notably that of the amenorrhea criterion being removed. Amenorrhea was removed for several reasons: it does not apply to males, it is not applicable for females before or after the age of menstruation or taking birth control pills, and some women who meet the other criteria for AN still report some menstrual activity.

Subtypes

There are two subtypes of AN:

- Binge-eating/purging type: the individual utilizes binge eating or displays purging behavior as a means for losing weight. It is different from bulimia nervosa in terms of the individual's weight. An individual with binge-eating/purging type anorexia can maintain a healthy or normal weight, but is usually significantly underweight. People with bulimia nervosa on the other hand can sometimes be overweight.

- Restricting type: the individual uses restricting food intake, fasting, diet pills, or exercise as a means for losing weight; they may exercise excessively to keep off weight or prevent weight gain, and some individuals eat only enough to stay alive.

Levels of Severity

Body mass index (BMI) is used by the DSM-5 as an indicator of the level of severity of anorexia nervosa. The DSM-5 states these as follows:

- Mild: BMI of greater than 17

- Moderate: BMI of 16–16.99

- Severe: BMI of 15–15.99

- Extreme: BMI of less than 15

Investigations

Medical tests to check for signs of physical deterioration in anorexia nervosa may be performed by a general physician or psychiatrist, including:

- Complete Blood Count (CBC): a test of the white blood cells, red blood cells and platelets used to assess the presence of various disorders such as leukocytosis, leukopenia, thrombocytosis and anemia which may result from malnutrition.

- Urinalysis: a variety of tests performed on the urine used in the diagnosis of medical disorders, to test for substance abuse, and as an indicator of overall health

- Chem-20: Chem-20 also known as SMA-20 a group of twenty separate chemical tests performed on blood serum. Tests include cholesterol, protein and electrolytes such as potassium, chlorine and sodium and tests specific to liver and kidney function.

- Glucose tolerance test: Oral glucose tolerance test (OGTT) used to assess the body's ability to metabolize glucose. Can be useful in detecting various disorders such as diabetes, an insulinoma, Cushing's Syndrome, hypoglycemia and polycystic ovary syndrome.

- Serum cholinesterase test: a test of liver enzymes (acetylcholinesterase and pseudocholinesterase) useful as a test of liver function and to assess the effects of malnutrition.

- Liver Function Test: A series of tests used to assess liver function some of the tests are also used in the assessment of malnutrition, protein deficiency, kidney function, bleeding disorders, and Crohn's Disease.

- Lh response to GnRH: Luteinizing hormone (Lh) response to gonadotropin-releasing hormone (GnRH): Tests the pituitary glands' response to GnRh a hormone produced in the hypothalamus. Hypogonadism is often seen in anorexia nervosa cases.

- Creatine Kinase Test (CK-Test): measures the circulating blood levels of creatine kinase an enzyme found in the heart (CK-MB), brain (CK-BB) and skeletal muscle (CK-MM).

- Blood urea nitrogen (BUN) test: urea nitrogen is the byproduct of protein metabolism first formed in the liver then removed from the body by the kidneys. The BUN test is primarily used to test kidney function. A low BUN level may indicate the effects of malnutrition.

- BUN-to-creatinine ratio: A BUN to creatinine ratio is used to predict various conditions. A high BUN/creatinine ratio can occur in severe hydration, acute kidney failure, congestive heart failure, and intestinal bleeding. A low BUN/creatinine ratio can indicate a low protein diet, celiac disease, rhabdomyolysis, or cirrhosis of the liver.

- Electrocardiogram (EKG or ECG): measures electrical activity of the heart. It can be used to detect various disorders such as hyperkalemia

- Electroencephalogram (EEG): measures the electrical activity of the brain. It can be used to detect abnormalities such as those associated with pituitary tumors.

- Thyroid Screen TSH, t4, t3 :test used to assess thyroid functioning by checking levels of thyroid-stimulating hormone (TSH), thyroxine (T4), and triiodothyronine (T3)

Differential Diagnoses

A variety of medical and psychological conditions have been misdiagnosed as anorexia nervosa; in some cases the correct diagnosis was not made for more than ten years.

The distinction between the diagnoses of anorexia nervosa, bulimia nervosa and eating disorder not otherwise specified (EDNOS) is often difficult to make as there is considerable overlap between people diagnosed with these conditions. Seemingly minor changes in a people's overall behavior or attitude can change a diagnosis from anorexia: binge-eating type to bulimia nervosa.

A main factor differentiating binge-purge anorexia from bulimia is the gap in physical weight. Someone with bulimia nervosa is ordinarily at a healthy weight, or slightly overweight. Someone with binge-purge anorexia is commonly underweight. People with the binge-purging subtype of AN may be significantly underweight and typically do not binge-eat large amounts of food, yet they purge the small amount of food they eat. In contrast, those with bulimia nervosa tend to be at normal weight or overweight and binge large amounts of food. It is not unusual for a person with an eating disorder to "move through" various diagnoses as their behavior and beliefs change over time.

Treatment

There is no conclusive evidence that any particular treatment for anorexia nervosa works better than others; however, there is enough evidence to suggest that early intervention and treatment are more effective. Treatment for anorexia nervosa tries to address three main areas.

- Restoring the person to a healthy weight;

- Treating the psychological disorders related to the illness;

- Reducing or eliminating behaviours or thoughts that originally led to the disordered eating.

Although restoring the person's weight is the primary task at hand, optimal treatment also includes and monitors behavioral change in the individual as well. There is some evidence that hospitalisation might adversely affect long term outcome.

Psychotherapy for individuals with AN is challenging as they may value being thin and may seek to maintain control and resist change. Some studies demonstrate that family based therapy in adolescents with AN is superior to individual therapy.

Treatment of people with AN is difficult because they are afraid of gaining weight. Initially developing a desire to change may be important.

Diet

Diet is the most essential factor to work on in people with anorexia nervosa, and must be tailored to each person's needs. Food variety is important when establishing meal plans as well as foods that are higher in energy density. People must consume adequate calories, starting slowly, and increasing at a measured pace. Evidence of a role for zinc supplementation during refeeding is unclear.

Therapy

Family-based treatment (FBT) has been shown to be more successful than individual therapy for adolescents with AN. Various forms of family-based treatment have been proven to work in the treatment of adolescent AN including conjoint family therapy (CFT), in which the parents and child are seen together by the same therapist, and separated family therapy (SFT) in which the parents and child attend therapy separately with different therapists. Proponents of Family therapy for adolescents with AN assert that it is important to include parents in the adolescent's treatment.

A four- to five-year follow up study of the Maudsley family therapy, an evidence-based manualized model, showed full recovery at rates up to 90%. Although this model is recommended by the NIMH, critics claim that it has the potential to create power struggles in an intimate relationship and may disrupt equal partnerships.

Cognitive behavioral therapy (CBT) is useful in adolescents and adults with anorexia nervosa; acceptance and commitment therapy is a type of CBT, which has shown promise in the treatment of AN. Cognitive remediation therapy (CRT) is used in treating anorexia nervosa.

Medication

Pharmaceuticals have limited benefit for anorexia itself.

Admission to Hospital

AN has a high mortality and patients admitted in a severely ill state to medical units are at particularly high risk. Diagnosis can be challenging, risk assessment may not be performed accurately, consent and the need for compulsion may not be assessed appropriately, refeeding syndrome may be missed or poorly treated and the behavioural and family problems in AN may be missed or poorly managed. The MARSIPAN guidelines recommend that medical and psychiatric experts work together in managing severely ill people with AN.

Nutrition

The rate of refeeding can be difficult to establish, because the fear of refeeding syndrome (RFS) can lead to underfeeding. It is thought that RFS, with falling phosphate and potassium levels, is more likely to occur when BMI is very low, and when medical comorbidities such as infection or cardiac failure, are present. In those circumstances, it is recommended to start refeeding slowly but to build up rapidly as long as RFS does not occur. Recommendations on energy requirements vary, from 5–10 kCal/Kg/day in the most medically compromised patients, who appear to have the highest risk of RFS to 1900 Kcal/day.

Prognosis

AN has the highest mortality rate of any psychological disorder. The mortality rate is 11 to 12 times greater than in the general population, and the suicide risk is 56 times higher. Half of women with AN achieve a full recovery, while an additional 20–30% may partially recover. Not all people with anorexia recover completely: about 20% develop anorexia nervosa as a chronic disorder. If anorexia nervosa is not treated, serious complications such as heart conditions and kidney failure can arise and eventually lead to death. The average number of years from onset to remission of AN is seven for women and three for men. After ten to fifteen years, 70% of people no longer meet the diagnostic criteria, but many still continue to have eating-related problems.

Alexithymia influences treatment outcome. Recovery is also viewed on a spectrum rather than black and white. According to the Morgan-Russell criteria, individuals can have a good, intermediate, or poor outcome. Even when a person is classified as having a "good" outcome, weight only has to be within 15% of average, and normal menstruation must be present in females. The good outcome also excludes psychological health. Recovery for people with anorexia nervosa is undeniably positive, but recovery does not mean a return to normal.

Complications

Anorexia nervosa can have serious implications if its duration and severity are significant and if onset occurs before the completion of growth, pubertal maturation, or the attainment of peak bone mass. Complications specific to adolescents and children with anorexia nervosa can include the following: Growth retardation may occur, as height gain may slow and can stop completely with severe weight loss or chronic malnutrition. In such cases, provided that growth potential is preserved, height increase can resume and reach full potential after normal intake is resumed. Height potential is normally preserved if the duration and severity of illness are not significant or if the illness is accompanied by delayed bone age (especially prior to a bone age of approximately 15 years), as hypogonadism may partially counteract the effects of undernutrition on height by allowing for a longer duration of growth compared to controls. Appropriate early treatment can preserve height potential, and may even help to increase it in some post-anorexic subjects, due to factors such as long-term reduced estrogen-producing adipose tissue levels compared to premorbid levels. In some cases, especially where onset is before puberty, complications such as stunted growth and pubertal delay are usually reversible.

Anorexia nervosa causes alterations in the female reproductive system; significant weight loss, as well as psychological stress and intense exercise, typically results in a cessation of menstruation in women who are past puberty. In patients with anorexia nervosa, there is a reduction of the secretion of gonadotropin releasing hormone in the central nervous system, preventing ovulation. Anorexia nervosa can also result in pubertal delay or arrest. Both height gain and pubertal development are dependent on the release of growth hormone and gonadotrophins (LH and FSH) from the pituitary gland. Suppression of gonadotrophins in people with anorexia nervosa has been documented. Typically, growth hormone (GH) levels are high, but levels of IGF-1, the downstream hormone that should be released in response to GH are low; this indicates a state of "resistance" to GH due to chronic starvation. IGF-1 is necessary for bone formation, and decreased levels in anorexia nervosa contribute to a loss of bone density and potentially contribute to osteopenia or osteoporosis. Anorexia nervosa can also result in reduction of peak bone mass. Buildup of bone is greatest during adolescence, and if onset of anorexia nervosa occurs during this time and stalls puberty, low bone mass may be permanent. Hepatic steatosis, or fatty infiltration of the liver, can also occur, and is an indicator of malnutrition in children. Neurological disorders that may occur as complications include seizures and tremors. Wernicke encephalopathy, which results from vitamin B1 deficiency, has been reported in patients who are extremely malnourished; symptoms include confusion, problems with the muscles responsible for eye movements and abnormalities in walking gait.

The most common gastrointestinal complications of anorexia nervosa are delayed stomach emptying and constipation, but also include elevated liver function tests, diarrhea, acute pancreatitis, heartburn, difficulty swallowing, and, rarely, superior mesenteric artery syndrome. Delayed stomach emptying, or gastroparesis, often develops following food restriction and weight loss; the most common symptom is bloating with gas and abdominal distension, and often occurs after eating. Other symptoms of gastroparesis include early satiety, fullness, nausea, and vomiting. The symptoms may inhibit efforts at eating and recovery, but can be managed by limiting high-fiber foods, using liquid nutritional supplements, or using metoclopramide to increase emptying of food from the stomach. Gastroparesis generally resolves when weight is regained.

Cardiac Complications

Anorexia nervosa increases the risk of sudden cardiac death, though the precise cause is unknown. Cardiac complications include structural and functional changes to the heart. Some of these cardiovascular changes are mild and are reversible with treatment, while others may be life-threatening. Cardiac complications can include arrhythmias, abnormally slow heart beat, low blood pressure, decreased size of the heart muscle, reduced heart volume, mitral valve prolapse, myocardial fibrosis, and pericardial effusion.

Abnormalities in conduction and repolarization of the heart that can result from anorexia nervosa include QT prolongation, increased QT dispersion, conduction delays, and junctional escape rhythms. Electrolyte abnormalities, particularly hypokalemia and hypomagnesemia, can cause anomalies in the electrical activity of the heart, and result in life-threatening arrhythmias. Hypokalemia most commonly results in anorexic patients when restricting is accompanied by purging (induced vomiting or laxative use). Hypotension (low blood pressure) is common, and symptoms include fatigue and weakness. Orthostatic hypotension, a marked decrease in blood pressure when standing from a supine position, may also occur. Symptoms include lightheadedness upon standing, weakness, and cognitive impairment, and may result in fainting or near-fainting. Orthostasis in anorexia nervosa indicates worsening cardiac function and may indicate a need for hospitalization. Hypotension and orthostasis generally resolve upon recovery to a normal weight. The weight loss in anorexia nervosa also causes atrophy of cardiac muscle. This leads to decreased ability to pump blood, a reduction in the ability to sustain exercise, a diminished ability to increase blood pressure in response to exercise, and a subjective feeling of fatigue. Some individuals may also have a decrease in cardiac contractility. Cardiac complications can be life-threatening, but the heart muscle generally improves with weight gain, and the heart normalizes in size normalizes over weeks to months, with recovery. Atrophy of the heart muscle is a marker of the severity of the disease, and while it is reversible with treatment and refeeding, it is possible that it may cause permanent, microscopic changes to the heart muscle that increase the risk of sudden cardiac death. Individuals with anorexia nervosa may experience chest pain or palpitations; these can be a result of mitral valve prolapse. Mitral valve prolapse occurs because the size of the heart muscle decreases while the tissue of the mitral valve remains the same size. Studies have shown rates of mitral valve prolapse of around 20 percent in those with anorexia nervosa, while the rate in the general population is estimated at 2–4 percent. It has been suggested that there is an association between mitral valve prolapse and sudden cardiac death, but it has not been proven to be causative, either in patients with anorexia nervosa or in the general population.

Relapse

Relapse occurs in approximately a third of people in hospital, and is greatest in the first six to eighteen months after release from an institution.

Epidemiology

Anorexia is estimated to occur in 0.9% to 4.3% of women and 0.2% to 0.3% of men in Western countries at some point in their life. About 0.4% of young females are affected in a given year and it is estimated to occur three to ten times less commonly in males. Rates in most of the developing world are unclear. Often it begins during the teen years or young adulthood.

The lifetime rate of atypical anorexia nervosa, a form of ED-NOS in which not all of the diagnostic criteria for AN are met, is much higher, at 5–12%.

While anorexia become more commonly diagnosed during the 20th century it is unclear if this was due to an increase in its frequency or simply better diagnosis. Most studies show that since at least 1970 the incidence of AN in adult women is fairly constant, while there is some indication that the incidence may have been increasing for girls aged between 14 and 20.

Underrepresentation

Eating disorders are less reported in preindustrial, non-westernized countries than in Western countries. In Africa, not including South Africa, the only data presenting information about eating disorders occurs in case reports and isolated studies, not studies investigating prevalence. Data shows in research that in westernized civilizations, ethnic minorities have very similar rates of eating disorders, contrary to the belief that eating disorders predominantly occur in Caucasian people.

Due to different standards of beauty for men and women, men are often not diagnosed as anorexic. Generally men who alter their bodies do so to be lean and muscular rather than thin. In addition, men who might otherwise be diagnosed with anorexia may not meet the DSM IV criteria for BMI since they have muscle weight, but have very little fat. Men and women athletes are often overlooked as anorexic. Research emphasizes the importance to take athletes' diet, weight and symptoms into account when diagnosing anorexia, instead of just looking at weight and BMI. For athletes, ritualized activities such as weigh-ins place emphasis on weight, which may promote the development of eating disorders among them. While women use diet pills, which is an indicator of unhealthy behavior and an eating disorder, men use steroids, which contextualizes the beauty ideals for genders. This also shows men having a preoccupation with their body, which is an indicator of an eating disorder. In a Canadian study, 4% of boys in grade nine used anabolic steroids. Anorexic men are sometimes referred to as *manorexic*.

History

The term *anorexia nervosa* was coined in 1873 by Sir William Gull, one of Queen Victoria's personal physicians. The history of anorexia nervosa begins with descriptions of religious fasting dating from the Hellenistic era and continuing into the medieval period. The medieval practice of self-starvation by women, including some young women, in the name of religious piety and purity also concerns anorexia nervosa; it is sometimes referred to as *anorexia mirabilis*.

The earliest medical descriptions of anorexic illnesses are generally credited to English physician Richard Morton in 1689. Case descriptions fitting anorexic illnesses continued throughout the 17th, 18th and 19th centuries.

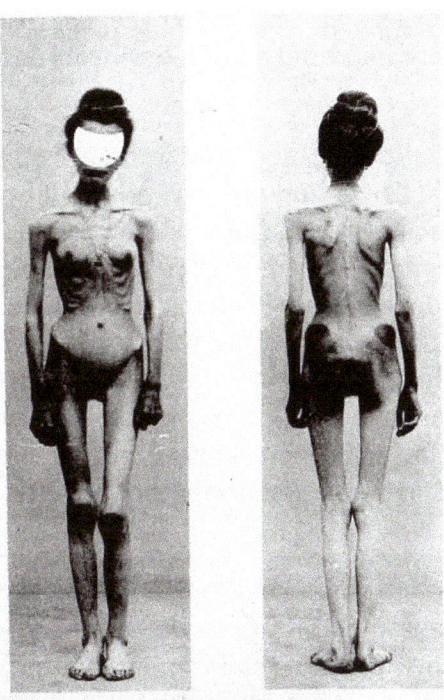

Two images of an anorexic female published in 1900 in
"Nouvelle Iconographie de la Salpêtrière". The case was entitiled
"Un cas d'anorexie hysterique" (A case of hysteria anorexia).

In the late 19th century anorexia nervosa became widely accepted by the medical profession as a recognized condition. In 1873, Sir William Gull, one of Queen Victoria's personal physicians, published a seminal paper which coined the term *anorexia nervosa* and provided a number of detailed case descriptions and treatments. In the same year, French physician Ernest-Charles Lasègue similarly published details of a number of cases in a paper entitled *De l'Anorexie hystérique*.

Awareness of the condition was largely limited to the medical profession until the latter part of the 20th century, when German-American psychoanalyst Hilde Bruch published *The Golden Cage: the Enigma of Anorexia Nervosa* in 1978. Despite major advances in neuroscience, Bruch's theories tend to dominate popular thinking. A further important event was the death of the popular singer and drummer Karen Carpenter in 1983, which prompted widespread ongoing media coverage of eating disorders.

Malnutrition

Malnutrition is a condition that results from eating a diet in which nutrients are either not enough or are too much such that the diet causes health problems. It may involve calories, protein, carbohydrates, vitamins or minerals. Not enough nutrients is called undernutrition or undernourishment while too much is called overnutrition. Malnutrition is often used to specifically refer to undernutrition where an individual is not getting enough calories, protein, or micronutrients. If undernutrition occurs during pregnancy, or before two years of age, it may result in permanent problems with physical and mental development. Extreme undernourishment, known as starvation, may have symptoms that include: a short height, thin body, very poor energy levels, and swollen legs and abdomen. People also often get infections and are frequently cold. The symptoms of micronutrient deficiencies depend on the micronutrient that is lacking.

Undernourishment is most often due to not enough high-quality food being available to eat. This is often related to high food prices and poverty. A lack of breastfeeding may contribute, as may a number of infectious diseases such as: gastroenteritis, pneumonia, malaria, and measles, which increase nutrient requirements. There are two main types of undernutrition: protein-energy malnutrition and dietary deficiencies. Protein-energy malnutrition has two severe forms: marasmus (a lack of protein and calories) and kwashiorkor (a lack of just protein). Common micronutrient deficiencies include: a lack of iron, iodine, and vitamin A. During pregnancy, due to the body's increased need, deficiencies may become more common. In some developing countries, overnutrition in the form of obesity is beginning to present within the same communities as undernutrition. Other causes of malnutrition include anorexia nervosa and bariatric surgery.

Efforts to improve nutrition are some of the most effective forms of development aid. Breastfeeding can reduce rates of malnutrition and death in children, and efforts to promote the practice increase the rates of breastfeeding. In young children, providing food (in addition to breastmilk) between six months and two years of age improves outcomes. There is also good evidence supporting the supplementation of a number of micronutrients to women during pregnancy and among young children in the developing world. To get food to people who need it most, both delivering food and providing money so people can buy food within local markets are effective. Simply feeding students at school is insufficient. Management of severe malnutrition within the person's home with ready-to-use therapeutic foods is possible much of the time. In those who have severe malnutrition complicated by other health problems, treatment in a hospital setting is recommended. This often involves managing low blood sugar and body temperature, addressing dehydration, and gradual feeding. Routine antibiotics are usually recommended due to the high risk of infection. Longer-term measures include: improving agricultural practices, reducing poverty, improving sanitation, and the empowerment of women.

There were 793 million undernourished people in the world in 2015 (13% of the total population). This is a reduction of 216 million people since 1990 when 23% were undernourished. In 2012 it was estimated that another billion people had a lack of vitamins and minerals. In 2015, protein-energy malnutrition was estimated to have resulted in 323,000 deaths—down from 510,000 deaths in 1990. Other nutritional deficiencies, which include iodine deficiency and iron deficiency anemia, result in another 83,000 deaths. In 2010, malnutrition was the cause of 1.4% of all disability adjusted life years. About a third of deaths in children are believed to be due to undernutrition, although the deaths are rarely labelled as such. In 2010, it was estimated to have contributed to about 1.5 million deaths in women and children, though some estimate the number may be greater than 3 million. An additional 165 million children were estimated to have stunted growth from malnutrition in 2013. Undernutrition is more common in developing countries. Certain groups have higher rates of undernutrition, including women—in particular while pregnant or breastfeeding—children under five years of age, and the elderly. In the elderly, undernutrition becomes more common due to physical, psychological, and social factors.

Definitions

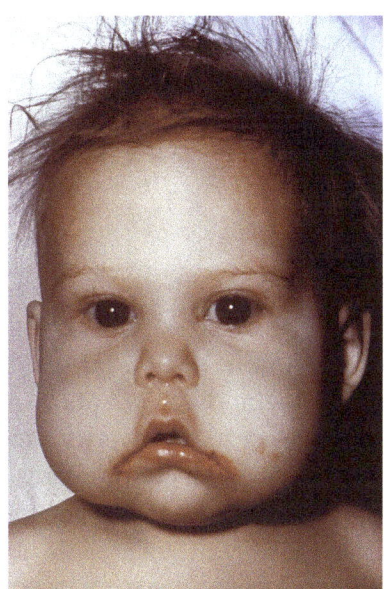

Child in the United States with signs of Kwashiorkor, a dietary protein deficiency.

Unless specifically mentioned otherwise, the term malnutrition refers to undernutrition for the remainder of this article. Malnutrition can be divided into two different types, SAM and MAM. SAM refers to children with severe acute malnutrition. MAM refers to moderate acute malnutrition.

Undernutrition and Overnutrition

Malnutrition is caused by eating a diet in which nutrients are *not enough* or are *too much* such that it causes health problems. It is a category of diseases that includes undernutrition and overnutrition. Overnutrition can result in obesity and being overweight. In some developing countries, overnutrition in the form of obesity is beginning to present within the same communities as undernutrition.

However, the term malnutrition is commonly used to refer to undernutrition only. This applies particularly to the context of development cooperation. Therefore, "malnutrition" in documents by the World Health Organization, UNICEF, Save the Children or other international non-governmental organizations (NGOs) usually is equated to undernutrition.

Protein-energy Malnutrition

Undernutrition is sometimes used as a synonym of protein–energy malnutrition (PEM). While other include both micronutrient deficiencies and protein energy malnutrition in its definition. It differs from calorie restriction in that calorie restriction may not result in negative health effects. The term hypoalimentation means underfeeding.

The term "severe malnutrition" or "severe undernutrition" is often used to refer specifically to PEM. PEM is often associated with micronutrient deficiency. Two forms of PEM are kwashiorkor and marasmus, and they commonly coexist.

Kwashiorkor

Kwashiorkor ('displaced child') is mainly caused by inadequate protein intake resulting in a low concentration of amino acids. The main symptoms are edema, wasting, liver enlargement, hypoalbuminaemia, steatosis, and possibly depigmentation of skin and hair. Kwashiorkor is identified by swelling of the extremities and belly, which is deceiving of actual nutritional status.

Marasmus

Marasmus ('to waste away') is caused by an inadequate intake of protein and energy. The main symptoms are severe wasting, leaving little or no edema, minimal subcutaneous fat, severe muscle wasting, and non-normal serum albumin levels. Marasmus can result from a sustained diet of inadequate energy and protein, and the metabolism adapts to prolong survival. It is traditionally seen in famine, significant food restriction, or more severe cases of anorexia. Conditions are characterized by extreme wasting of the muscles and a gaunt expression.

Undernutrition, Hunger

Undernutrition encompasses stunted growth (stunting), wasting, and deficiencies of essential vitamins and minerals (collectively referred to as micronutrients). The term hunger, which describes a feeling of discomfort from not eating, has been used to describe undernutrition, especially in reference to food insecurity.

Definition by Gomez

In 1956, Gómez and Galvan studied factors associated with death in a group of malnourished (undernourished) children in a hospital in Mexico City, Mexico and defined categories of malnutrition: first, second, and third degree. The degrees were based on weight below a specified percentage of median weight for age. The risk of death increases with increasing degree of malnutrition. An adaptation of Gomez's original classification is still used today. While it provides a way to compare malnutrition within and between populations, the classification has been criticized for being "arbitrary" and for not considering overweight as a form of malnutrition. Also, height alone may not be the best indicator of malnutrition; children who are born prematurely may be considered short for their age even if they have good nutrition.

Degree of PEM	% of Desired Body Weight for Age and Sex
Normal	90%-100%
Mild: Grade I (1st degree)	75%-89%
Moderate: Grade II (2nd degree)	60%-74%
Severe: Grade III (3rd degree)	<60%
SOURCE:"Serum Total Protein and Albumin Levels in Different Grades of Protein Energy Malnutrition"	

Definition by Waterlow

John Conrad Waterlow established a new classification for malnutrition. Instead of using just weight for age measurements, the classification established by Waterlow combines weight-for-height (indicating acute episodes of malnutrition) with height-for-age to show the stunting that results from chronic malnutrition. One advantage of the Waterlow classification over the Gomez classification is that weight for height can be examined even if ages are not known.

Degree of PEM	Stunting (%) Height for age	Wasting (%) Weight for height
Normal: Grade 0	>95%	>90%
Mild: Grade I	87.5-95%	80-90%
Moderate: Grade II	80-87.5%	70-80%
Severe: Grade III	<80%	<70%
SOURCE: "Classification and definition of protein-calorie malnutrition." by Waterlow, 1972		

These classifications of malnutrition are commonly used with some modifications by WHO.

Effects

Malnutrition increases the risk of infection and infectious disease, and moderate malnutrition weakens every part of the immune system. For example, it is a major risk factor in the onset of active tuberculosis. Protein and energy malnutrition and deficiencies of specific micronutrients (including iron, zinc, and vitamins) increase susceptibility to infection. Malnutrition affects HIV transmission by increasing the risk of transmission from mother to child and also increasing replication of the virus. In communities or areas that lack access to safe drinking water, these additional health risks present a critical problem. Lower energy and impaired function of the brain also represent the downward spiral of malnutrition as victims are less able to perform the tasks they need to in order to acquire food, earn an income, or gain an education.

Vitamin-deficiency-related diseases (such as scurvy and rickets).

Hypoglycemia (low blood sugar) can result from a child not eating for 4 to 6 hours. Hypoglycemia should be considered if there is lethargy, limpness, convulsion, or loss of consciousness. If blood sugar can be measured immediately and quickly, perform a finger or heel stick.

Signs

In those with malnutrition some of the signs of dehydration differ. Children; however, may still be interested in drinking, have decreased interactions with the world around them, have decreased urine output, and may be cool to touch.

Site	Sign
Face	Moon face (kwashiorkor), simian facies (marasmus)
Eye	Dry eyes, pale conjunctiva, Bitot's spots (vitamin A), periorbital edema
Mouth	Angular stomatitis, cheilitis, glossitis, spongy bleeding gums (vitamin C), parotid enlargement
Teeth	Enamel mottling, delayed eruption
Hair	Dull, sparse, brittle hair, hypopigmentation, flag sign (alternating bands of light and normal color), broomstick eyelashes, alopecia
Skin	Loose and wrinkled (marasmus), shiny and edematous (kwashiorkor), dry, follicular hyperkeratosis, patchy hyper- and hypopigmentation, erosions, poor wound healing
Nail	Koilonychia, thin and soft nail plates, fissures or ridges
Musculature	Muscles wasting, particularly in the buttocks and thighs
Skeletal	Deformities usually a result of calcium, vitamin D, or vitamin C deficiencies
Abdomen	Distended - hepatomegaly with fatty liver, ascites may be present
Cardiovascular	Bradycardia, hypotension, reduced cardiac output, small vessel vasculopathy
Neurologic	Global development delay, loss of knee and ankle reflexes, poor memory
Hematological	Pallor, petechiae, bleeding diathesis
Behavior	Lethargic, apathetic
Source: "Protein Energy Malnutrition"	

Cognitive Development

Protein-calorie malnutrition can cause cognitive impairments. For humans, "critical period varies from the final third of gestation to the first 2 years of life". Iron deficiency anemia in children under two years of age likely affects brain function acutely and probably also chronically. Folate deficiency has been linked to neural tube defects.

Malnutrition in the form of iodine deficiency is "the most common preventable cause of mental impairment worldwide." "Even moderate deficiency, especially in pregnant women and infants, lowers intelligence by 10 to 15 I.Q. points, shaving incalculable potential off a nation's development. The most visible and severe effects — disabling goiters, cretinism and dwarfism — affect a tiny minority, usually in mountain villages. But 16 percent of the world's people have at least mild goiter, a swollen thyroid gland in the neck."

Causes

Major causes of malnutrition include poverty and food prices, dietary practices and agricultural productivity, with many individual cases being a mixture of several factors. Clinical malnutrition, such as in cachexia, is a major burden also in developed countries. Various scales of analysis also have to be considered in order to determine the sociopolitical causes of malnutrition. For example, the population of a community may be at risk if the area lacks health-related services, but on a smaller scale certain households or individuals may be at even higher risk due to differences in income levels, access to land, or levels of education.

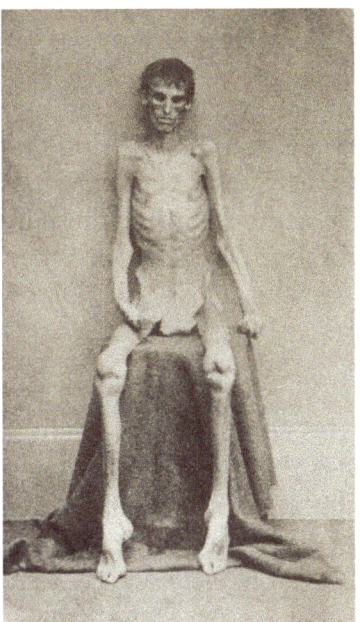

Union Army soldier on his release from Andersonville prison, 1865.

Diseases

Malnutrition can be a consequence of health issues such as gastroenteritis or chronic illness, especially the HIV/AIDS pandemic. Diarrhea and other infections can cause malnutrition through decreased nutrient absorption, decreased intake of food, increased metabolic requirements, and direct nutrient loss. Parasite infections, in particular intestinal worm infections (helminthiasis), can also lead to malnutrition. A leading cause of diarrhea and intestinal worm infections in children in developing countries is lack of sanitation and hygiene.

People may become malnourished due to abnormal nutrient loss (due to diarrhea or chronic illness affecting the small bowel). This conditions may include Crohn's disease or untreated coeliac disease. Malnutrition may also occur due to increased energy expenditure (secondary malnutrition).

Dietary Practices

Undernutrition

A lack of adequate breastfeeding leads to malnutrition in infants and children, associated with the deaths of an estimated one million children annually. Illegal advertising of breast milk substitutes continues three decades after its 1981 prohibition under the *WHO International Code of Marketing Breast Milk Substitutes*.

Deriving too much of one's diet from a single source, such as eating almost exclusively corn or rice, can cause malnutrition. This may either be from a lack of education about proper nutrition, or from only having access to a single food source.

It is not just the total amount of calories that matters but specific nutritional deficiencies such as vitamin A deficiency, iron deficiency or zinc deficiency can also increase risk of death.

Overnutrition

Overnutrition caused by overeating is also a form of malnutrition. In the United States, more than half of all adults are now overweight — a condition that, like hunger, increases susceptibility to disease and disability, reduces worker productivity, and lowers life expectancy. Overeating is much more common in the United States, where for the majority of people, access to food is not an issue. Many parts of the world have access to a surplus of non-nutritious food, in addition to increased sedentary lifestyles. Yale psychologist Kelly Brownell calls this a "toxic food environment" where fat and sugar laden foods have taken precedence over healthy nutritious foods.

The issue in these developed countries is choosing the right kind of food. More fast food is consumed per capita in the United States than in any other country. The reason for this mass consumption of fast food is its affordability and accessibility. Often fast food, low in cost and nutrition, is high in calories and heavily promoted. When these eating habits are combined with increasingly urbanized, automated, and more sedentary lifestyles, it becomes clear why weight gain is difficult to avoid.

Not only does obesity occur in developed countries, problems are also occurring in developing countries in areas where income is on the rise. Overeating is also a problem in countries where hunger and poverty persist. In China, consumption of high-fat foods has increased while consumption of rice and other goods has decreased.

Overeating leads to many diseases, such as heart disease and diabetes, that may result in death.

Poverty and Food Prices

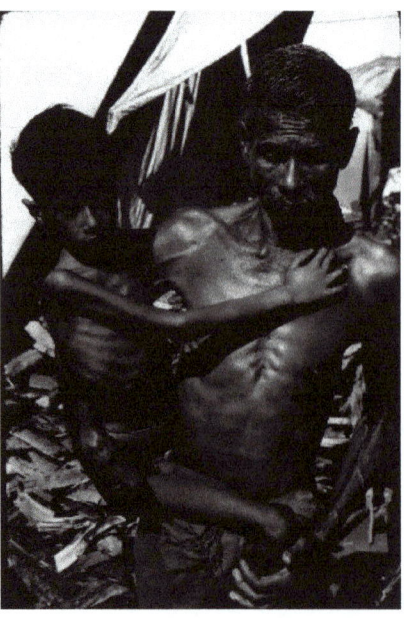

A child with extreme malnutrition

In Bangladesh, poor socioeconomic position was associated with chronic malnutrition since it inhibits purchase of nutritious foods such as milk, meat, poultry, and fruits. As much as food shortages may be a contributing factor to malnutrition in countries with lack of technology, the FAO (Food and Agriculture Organization) has estimated that eighty percent of malnourished children living in the developing world live in countries that produce food surpluses. The economist Amartya Sen observed that, in recent decades, famine has always been a problem of food distribution and/or poverty, as there has been sufficient food to feed the whole population of the world. He states that malnutrition and famine were more related to problems of food distribution and purchasing power.

It is argued that commodity speculators are increasing the cost of food. As the real estate bubble in the United States was collapsing, it is said that trillions of dollars moved to invest in food and primary commodities, causing the 2007–2008 food price crisis.

The use of biofuels as a replacement for traditional fuels and raises the price of food. The United Nations special rapporteur on the right to food, Jean Ziegler proposes that agricultural waste, such as corn cobs and banana leaves, rather than crops themselves be used as fuel.

Agricultural Productivity

Local food shortages can be caused by a lack of arable land, adverse weather, lower farming skills such as crop rotation, or by a lack of technology or resources needed for the higher yields found in modern agriculture, such as fertilizers, pesticides, irrigation, machinery and storage facilities. As a result of widespread poverty, farmers cannot afford or governments cannot provide the resources necessary to improve local yields. The World Bank and some wealthy donor countries also press nations that depend on aid to cut or eliminate subsidized agricultural inputs such as fertilizer, in the name of free market policies even as the United States and Europe extensively subsidized their own farmers. Many, if not most, farmers cannot afford fertilizer at market prices, leading to low agricultural production and wages and high, unaffordable food prices. Reasons for the unavailability of fertilizer include moves to stop supplying fertilizer on environmental grounds, cited as the obstacle to feeding Africa by the Green Revolution pioneers Norman Borlaug and Keith Rosenberg.

Future Threats

There are a number of potential disruptions to global food supply that could cause widespread malnutrition.

Climate change is of importance to food security, with 95 percent of all malnourished peoples living in the relatively stable climate region of the sub-tropics and tropics. According to the latest IPCC reports, temperature increases in these regions are "very likely." Even small changes in temperatures can lead to increased frequency of extreme weather conditions. Many of these have great impact on agricultural production and hence nutrition. For example, the 1998–2001 central Asian drought brought about an 80 percent livestock loss and 50 percent reduction in wheat and barley crops in Iran. Similar figures were present in other nations. An increase in extreme weather such as drought in regions such as Sub-Saharan Africa would have even greater consequences in terms of malnutrition. Even without an increase of extreme weather events, a simple increase in temperature reduces the productivity of many crop species, also decreasing food security in these regions.

Colony collapse disorder is a phenomenon where bees die in large numbers. Since many agricultural crops worldwide are pollinated by bees, this represents a threat to the supply of food.

An epidemic of wheat stem rust caused by race Ug99 is currently spreading across Africa and into Asia and, it is feared, could wipe out more than 80 percent of the world's wheat crops.

Prevention

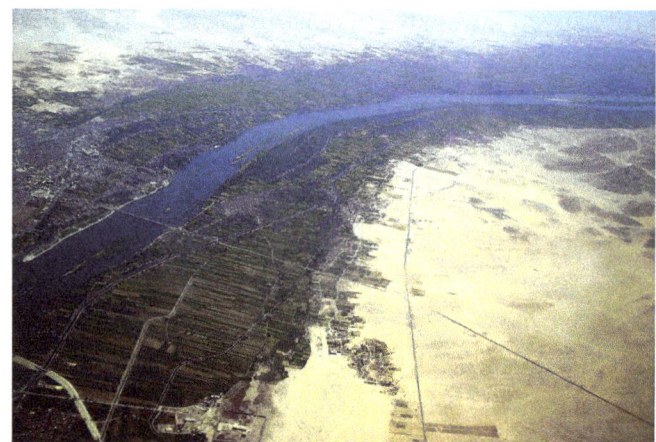

Irrigation canals have opened dry desert areas of Egypt to agriculture.

Food Security

The effort to bring modern agricultural techniques found in the West, such as nitrogen fertilizers and pesticides, to Asia, called the Green Revolution, resulted in decreases in malnutrition similar to those seen earlier in Western nations. This was possible because of existing infrastructure and institutions that are in short supply in Africa, such as a system of roads or public seed companies that made seeds available. Investments in agriculture, such as subsidized fertilizers and seeds, increases food harvest and reduces food prices. For example, in the case of Malawi, almost five million of its 13 million people used to need emergency food aid. However, after the government changed policy and subsidies for fertilizer and seed were introduced against World Bank strictures, farmers produced record-breaking corn harvests as production leaped to 3.4 million in 2007 from 1.2 million in 2005, making Malawi a major food exporter. This lowered food prices and increased wages for farm workers. Such investments in agriculture are still needed in other African countries like the Democratic Republic of the Congo. The country has one of the highest prevalence of malnutrition even though it is blessed with great agricultural potential John Ulimwengu explains in his article for D+C. Proponents for investing in agriculture include Jeffrey Sachs, who has championed the idea that wealthy countries should invest in fertilizer and seed for Africa's farmers.

New technology in agricultural production also has great potential to combat undernutrition. By improving agricultural yields, farmers could reduce poverty by increasing income as well as open up area for diversification of crops for household use. The World Bank itself claims to be part of the solution to malnutrition, asserting that the best way for countries to succeed in breaking the cycle of poverty and malnutrition is to build export-led economies that will give them the financial means to buy foodstuffs on the world market.

Breastfeeding

As of 2016 is estimated that about 821,000 deaths of children less than five years old could be prevented globally per year through more widespread breastfeeding.

Fortified Foods

Manufacturers are trying to fortify everyday foods with micronutrients that can be sold to consumers such as wheat flour for Beladi bread in Egypt or fish sauce in Vietnam and the iodization of salt.

For example, flour has been fortified with iron, zinc, folic acid and other B vitamins such as thiamine, riboflavin,niacin and vitamin B12.

World Population

Restricting population size is a proposed solution. Thomas Malthus argued that population growth could be controlled by natural disasters and voluntary limits through "moral restraint." Robert Chapman suggests that an intervention through government policies is a necessary ingredient of curtailing global population growth. However, there are many who believe that the world has more than enough resources to sustain its population. Instead, these theorists point to unequal distribution of resources and under- or unutilized arable land as the cause for malnutrition problems. For example, Amartya Sen advocates that, "no matter how a famine is caused, methods of breaking it call for a large supply of food in the public distribution system. This applies not only to organizing rationing and control, but also to undertaking work programmes and other methods of increasing purchasing power for those hit by shifts in exchange entitlements in a general inflationary situation."

Food Sovereignty

One suggested policy framework to resolve access issues is termed food sovereignty—the right of peoples to define their own food, agriculture, livestock, and fisheries systems, in contrast to having food largely subjected to international market forces. Food First is one of the primary think tanks working to build support for food sovereignty. Neoliberals advocate for an increasing role of the free market.

Health Facilities

Another possible long term solution would be to increase access to health facilities to rural parts of the world. These facilities could monitor undernourished children, act as supplemental food distribution centers, and provide education on dietary needs. These types of facilities have already proven very successful in countries such as Peru and Ghana.

Global Initiatives

In April 2012, the Food Assistance Convention was signed, the world's first legally binding international agreement on food aid. The May 2012 Copenhagen Consensus recommended that efforts to combat hunger and malnutrition should be the first priority for politicians and private sector philanthropists looking to maximize the effectiveness of aid spending. They put this ahead of other priorities, like the fight against malaria and AIDS.

The main global policy to reduce hunger and poverty are the Sustainable Development Goals. In particular Goal 2: Zero hunger sets globally agreed targets to end hunger, achieve food security and improved nutrition and promote sustainable agriculture. The partnership Compact2025, led by IFPRI with the involvement of UN organisations, NGOs and private foundations develops and disseminates evidence-based advice to politicians and other decision-makers aimed at ending hunger and undernutrition in the coming 10 years, by 2025.

The EndingHunger campaign is an online communication campaign aimed at raising awareness of the hunger problem. It has many worked through viral videos depicting celebrities voicing their anger about the large number of hungry people in the world. Another initiative focused on improving the hunger situation by improving nutrition is the Scaling up Nutrition movement (SUN). Started in 2010 this movement of people from governments, civil society, the United Nations, donors, businesses and researchers, publishes a yearly progress report on the changes in their 55 partner countries.

Management

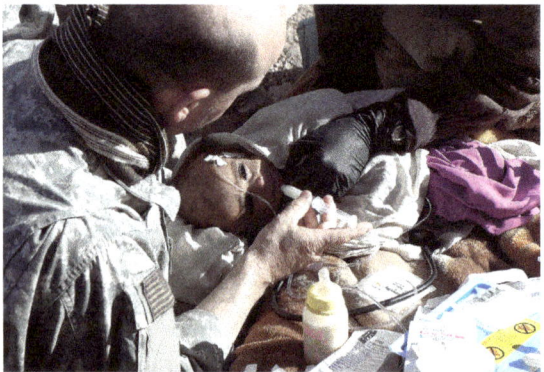

A malnourished Afghan child being treated by a medical team.

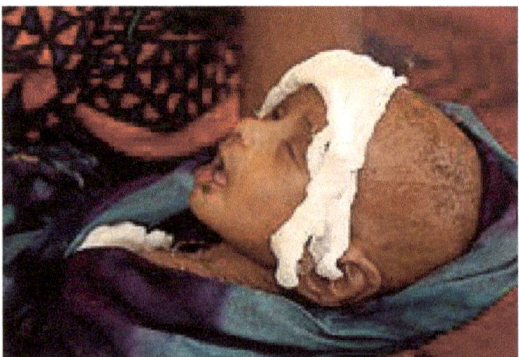

A Somali boy receiving treatment for malnourishment at a health facility.

In response to child malnutrition, the Bangladeshi government recommends ten steps for treating severe malnutrition. They are to prevent or treat dehydration, low blood sugar, low body temperature, infection, correct electrolyte imbalances and micronutrient deficiencies, start feeding cautiously, achieve catch-up growth, provide psychological support, and prepare for discharge and follow-up after recovery.

Among those patients who are hospitalized, nutritional support improves protein, colorie intake and weight.

Food

The evidence for benefit of supplementary feeding is poor. This is due to the small amount of research done on this treatment.

Specially formulated foods do however appear useful in those from the developing world with moderate acute malnutrition. In young children with severe acute malnutrition it is unclear if ready-to-use therapeutic food differs from a normal diet. They may have some benefits in humanitarian emergencies as they can be eaten directly from the packet, do not require refrigeration or mixing with clean water, and can be stored for years.

In those who are severely malnourished, feeding too much too quickly can result in refeeding syndrome. This can result regardless of route of feeding and can present itself a couple of days after eating with heart failure, dysrhythmias and confusion that can result in death.

Micronutrients

Treating malnutrition, mostly through fortifying foods with micronutrients (vitamins and minerals), improves lives at a lower cost and shorter time than other forms of aid, according to the World Bank. The Copenhagen Consensus, which look at a variety of development proposals, ranked micronutrient supplements as number one.

In those with diarrhea, once an initial four-hour rehydration period is completed, zinc supplementation is recommended. Daily zinc increases the chances of reducing the severity and duration of the diarrhea, and continuing with daily zinc for ten to fourteen days makes diarrhea less likely recur in the next two to three months.

In addition, malnourished children need both potassium and magnesium. This can be obtained by following the above recommendations for the dehydrated child to continue eating within two to three hours of starting rehydration, and including foods rich in potassium as above. Low blood potassium is worsened when base (as in Ringer's/Hartmann's) is given to treat acidosis without simultaneously providing potassium. As above, available home products such as salted and unsalted cereal water, salted and unsalted vegetable broth can be given early during the course of a child's diarrhea along with continued eating. Vitamin A, potassium, magnesium, and zinc should be added with other vitamins and minerals if available.

For a malnourished child with diarrhea from any cause, this should include foods rich in potassium such as bananas, green coconut water, and unsweetened fresh fruit juice.

Diarrhea

The World Health Organization (WHO) recommends rehydrating a severely undernourished child who has diarrhea relatively slowly. The preferred method is with fluids by mouth using a drink called oral rehydration solution (ORS). The oral rehydration solution is both slightly sweet and slightly salty and the one recommended in those with severe undernutrition should have half the usual sodium and greater potassium. Fluids by nasogastric tube may be use in those who do not drink. Intravenous fluids are recommended only in those who have significant dehydration due to their potential complications. These complications include congestive heart failure. Over time, ORS developed into ORT, or oral rehydration therapy, which focused on increasing fluids by supplying salts, carbohydrates, and water. This switch from type of fluid to amount of fluid was crucial in order to prevent dehydration from diarrhea.

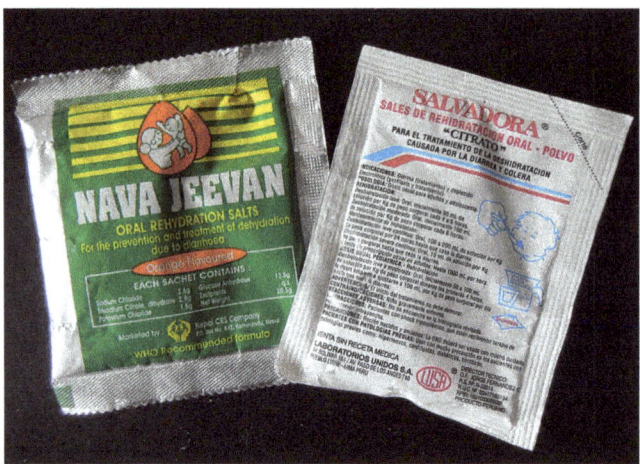

Examples of commercially available oral rehydration salts (Nepal on left, Peru on right).

Breast feeding and eating should resume as soon as possible. Drinks such as soft drinks, fruit juices, or sweetened teas are not recommended as they contain too much sugar and may worsen diarrhea. Broad spectrum antibiotics are recommended in all severely undernourished children with diarrhea requiring admission to hospital.

To prevent dehydration readily available fluids, preferably with a modest amount of sugars and salt such as vegetable broth or salted rice water, may be used. The drinking of additional clean water is also recommended. Once dehydration develops oral rehydration solutions are preferred. As much of these drinks as the person wants can be given, unless there are signs of swelling. If vomiting occurs, fluids can be paused for 5–10 minutes and then restarting more slowly. Vomiting rarely prevents rehydration as fluid are still absorbed and the vomiting rarely last long. A severely malnourished child with what appears to be dehydration but who has not had diarrhea should be treated as if they have an infection.

For babies a dropper or syringe without the needle can be used to put small amounts of fluid into the mouth; for children under 2, a teaspoon every one to two minutes; and for older children and adults, frequent sips directly from a cup. After the first two hours, rehydration should be continued at the same or slower rate, determined by how much fluid the child wants and any ongoing diarrheal loses. After the first two hours of rehydration it is recommended that to alternate between rehydration and food.

In 2003, WHO and UNICEF recommended a reduced-osmolarity ORS which still treats dehydration but also reduced stool volume and vomiting. Reduced-osmolarity ORS is the current standard

ORS with reasonably wide availability. For general use, one packet of ORS (glucose sugar, salt, potassium chloride, and trisodium citrate) is added to one liter of water; however, for malnourished children it is recommended that one packet of ORS be added to two liters of water along with an extra 50 grams of sucrose sugar and some stock potassium solution.

Malnourished children have an excess of body sodium. Recommendations for home remedies agree with one liter of water (34 oz.) and 6 teaspoons sugar and disagree regarding whether it is then one teaspoon of salt added or only 1/2, with perhaps most sources recommending 1/2 teaspoon of added salt to one liter water.

Low Blood Sugar

Hypoglycemia, whether known or suspected, can be treated with a mixture of sugar and water. If the child is conscious, the initial dose of sugar and water can be given by mouth. If the child is unconscious, give glucose by intravenous or nasogastric tube. If seizures occur after despite glucose, rectal diazepam is recommended. Blood sugar levels should be re-checked on two hour intervals.

Hypothermia

Hypothermia can occur. To prevent or treat this, the child can be kept warm with covering including of the head or by direct skin-to-skin contact with the mother or father and then covering both parent and child. Prolonged bathing or prolonged medical exams should be avoided. Warming methods are usually most important at night.

Economics

There is a growing realization among aid groups that giving cash or cash vouchers instead of food is a cheaper, faster, and more efficient way to deliver help to the hungry, particularly in areas where food is available but unaffordable. The UN's World Food Program, the biggest non-governmental distributor of food, announced that it will begin distributing cash and vouchers instead of food in some areas, which Josette Sheeran, the WFP's executive director, described as a "revolution" in food aid. The aid agency Concern Worldwide is piloting a method through a mobile phone operator, Safaricom, which runs a money transfer program that allows cash to be sent from one part of the country to another.

However, for people in a drought living a long way from and with limited access to markets, delivering food may be the most appropriate way to help. Fred Cuny stated that "the chances of saving lives at the outset of a relief operation are greatly reduced when food is imported. By the time it arrives in the country and gets to people, many will have died." U.S. law, which requires buying food at home rather than where the hungry live, is inefficient because approximately half of what is spent goes for transport. Cuny further pointed out "studies of every recent famine have shown that food was available in-country — though not always in the immediate food deficit area" and "even though by local standards the prices are too high for the poor to purchase it, it would usually be cheaper for a donor to buy the hoarded food at the inflated price than to import it from abroad."

Ethiopia has been pioneering a program that has now become part of the World Bank's prescribed method for coping with a food crisis and had been seen by aid organizations as a model of how to best help hungry nations. Through the country's main food assistance program, the Productive Safety Net Program, Ethiopia has been giving rural residents who are chronically short of food, a chance to work for food or cash. Foreign aid organizations like the World Food Program were then able to buy food locally from surplus areas to distribute in areas with a shortage of food. Ethiopia been pioneering a program, and Brazil has established a recycling program for organic waste that benefits farmers, urban poor, and the city in general. City residents separate organic waste from their garbage, bag it, and then exchange it for fresh fruit and vegetables from local farmers. As a result, the country's waste is reduced and the urban poor get a steady supply of nutritious food.

Epidemiology

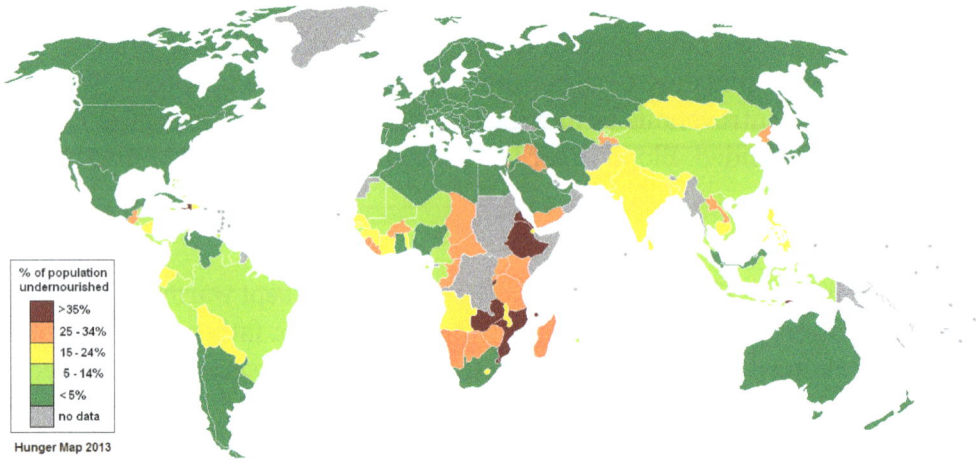

Percentage of population affected by undernutrition by country

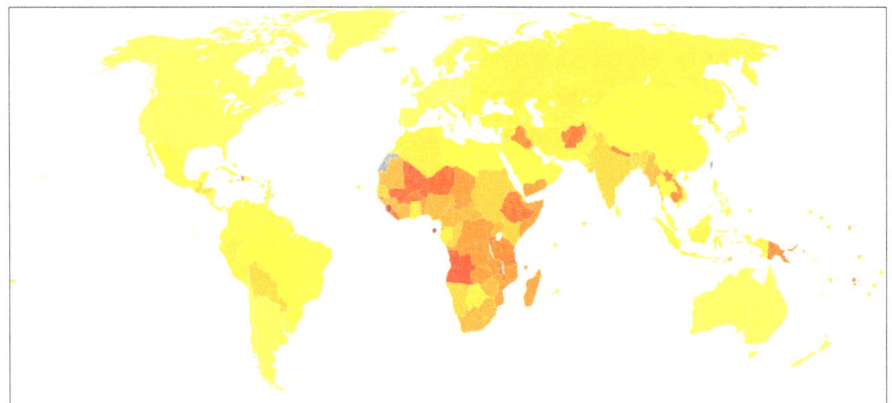

Disability-adjusted life year for nutritional deficiencies per 100,000 inhabitants in 2004. Nutritional deficiencies included: protein-energy malnutrition, iodine deficiency, vitamin A deficiency, and iron deficiency anaemia.

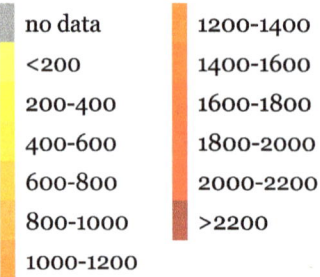

The figures provided in this section on epidemiology all refer to *undernutrition* even if the term malnutrition is used which, by definition, could also apply to too much nutrition.

People Affected

There were 793 million undernourished people in the world in 2015. This was 216 million fewer people than in 1990 when it was 991 million undernourished people. This is despite the world's farmers producing enough food to feed around 12 billion people – almost double the current world population.

Malnutrition, as of 2010, was the cause of 1.4% of all disability adjusted life years.

Number of UndernouriCshed Globally							
Year	1970	1980	1990	1995	2005	2007/08	2014/16
Number in millions			843	788	848	923	793
Percentage in the developing world	37%	28%	20%		16%	17%	13.5%

Mortality

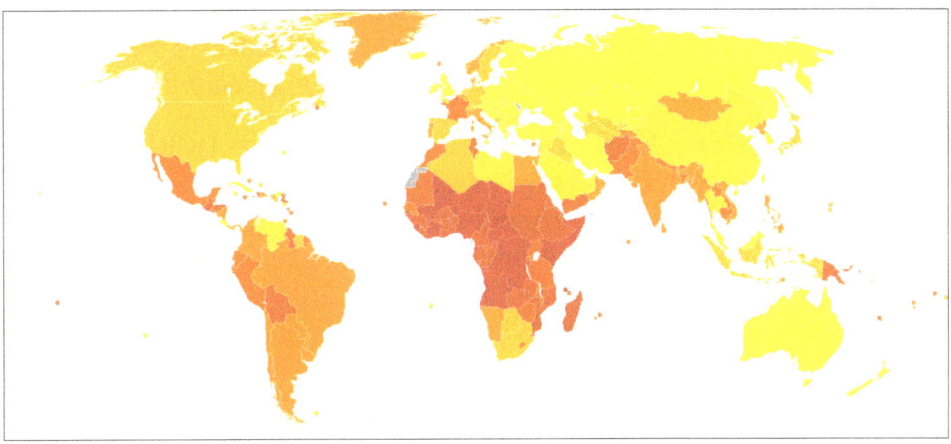

Deaths from nutritional deficiencies per million persons in 2012

	0-4
	5-8
	9-13
	14-23
	24-34
	35-56
	57-91
	92-220
	221-365
	366-1,207

Mortality due to malnutrition accounted for 58 percent of the total mortality in 2006: "In the world, approximately 62 million people, all causes of death combined, die each year. One in twelve people worldwide is malnourished and according to the Save the Children 2012 report, one in four of the world's children are chronically malnourished. In 2006, more than 36 million died of hunger or diseases due to deficiencies in micronutrients".

In 2010 protein-energy malnutrition resulted in 600,000 deaths down from 883,000 deaths in 1990. Other nutritional deficiencies, which include iodine deficiency and iron deficiency anemia, result in another 84,000 deaths. In 2010 malnutrition caused about 1.5 million deaths in women and children.

According to the World Health Organization, malnutrition is the biggest contributor to child mortality, present in half of all cases. Six million children die of hunger every year. Underweight births and intrauterine growth restrictions cause 2.2 million child deaths a year. Poor or non-existent breast-feeding causes another 1.4 million. Other deficiencies, such as lack of vitamin A or zinc, for example, account for 1 million. Malnutrition in the first two years is irreversible. Malnourished children grow up with worse health and lower education achievement. Their own children tend to be smaller. Malnutrition was previously seen as something that exacerbates the problems of diseases as measles, pneumonia and diarrhea. But malnutrition actually causes diseases and can be fatal in its own right.

Society and Culture

Roughly $300 million of aid goes to basic nutrition each year, less than $2 for each child below two in the 20 worst affected countries. In contrast, HIV/AIDS, which causes fewer deaths than child malnutrition, received $2.2 billion—$67 per person with HIV in all countries.

The International Crops Research Institute for the Semi-Arid Tropics (ICRISAT), a member of the CGIAR consortium, partners with farmers, governments, researchers and NGOs to help farmers grow nutritious crops, such as chickpea, groundnut, pigeonpea, millet and sorghum. This helps their communities have more balanced diets and become more resilient to pests and drought. The Harnessing Opportunities for Productivity Enhancement of Sorghum and Millets in Sub-Saharan Africa and the Indian-Subcontinent (HOPE) project, for example, is increasing yields of finger millet in Tanzania by encouraging farmers to grow improved varieties. Finger millet is very high in calcium, rich in iron and fiber, and has a better energy content than other cereals. These characteristics make it ideal for feeding to infants and the elderly.

Some organizations have begun working with teachers, policymakers, and managed food service contractors to mandate improved nutritional content and increased nutritional resources in school cafeterias from primary to university-level institutions. Health and nutrition have been proven to have close links with overall educational success.

The verb form is "malnourish"; "malnourishment" is sometimes used instead of "malnutrition."

Special Populations

Undernutrition is an important determinant of maternal and child health, accounting for more than a third of child deaths and more than 10 percent of the total global disease burden according to 2008 studies.

Children

The World Health Organization estimates that malnutrition accounts for 54 percent of child mortality worldwide, about 1 million children. Another estimate also by WHO states that childhood underweight is the cause for about 35% of all deaths of children under the age of five years worldwide.

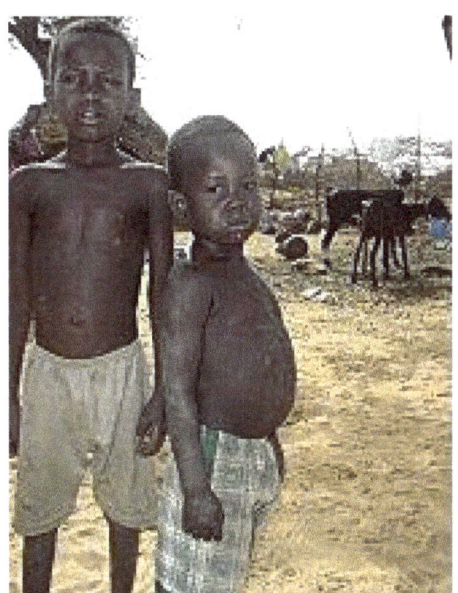

Malnourished children in Niger, during the 2005 famine.

As underweight children are more vulnerable to almost all infectious diseases, the *indirect* disease burden of malnutrition is estimated to be an order of magnitude higher than the disease burden of the *direct* effects of malnutrition. The combination of direct and indirect deaths from malnutrition caused by unsafe water, sanitation and hygiene (WASH) practices is estimated to lead to 860,000 deaths per year in children under five years of age.

Women

Gender

Researchers from the Centre for World Food Studies in 2003 found that the gap between levels of undernutrition in men and women is generally small, but that the gap varies from region to region and from country to country. These small-scale studies showed that female undernutrition prevalence rates exceeded male undernutrition prevalence rates in South/Southeast Asia and Latin America and were lower in Sub-Saharan Africa. Datasets for Ethiopia and Zimbabwe reported undernutrition rates between 1.5 and 2 times higher in men than in women; however, in India and Pakistan, datasets rates of undernutrition were 1.5-2 times higher in women than in men. Intra-country variation also occurs, with frequent high gaps between regional undernutrition rates. Gender inequality in nutrition in some countries such as India is present in all stages of life.

Studies on nutrition concerning gender bias within households look at patterns of food allocation, and one study from 2003 suggested that women often receive a lower share of food requirements than men. Gender discrimination, gender roles, and social norms affecting women can lead to early marriage and childbearing, close birth spacing, and undernutrition, all of which contribute to malnourished mothers.

Within the household, there may be differences in levels of malnutrition between men and women, and these differences have been shown to vary significantly from one region to another, with problem areas showing relative deprivation of women. Samples of 1000 women in India in 2008 demonstrated that malnutrition in women is associated with poverty, lack of development and awareness, and illiteracy. The same study showed that gender discrimination in households can prevent a woman's access to sufficient food and healthcare. How socialization affects the health of women in Bangladesh, Najma Rivzi explains in an article about a research program on this topic. In some cases, such as in parts of Kenya in 2006, rates of malnutrition in pregnant women were even higher than rates in children.

Women in some societies are traditionally given less food than men since men are perceived to have heavier workloads. Household chores and agricultural tasks can in fact be very arduous and require additional energy and nutrients; however, physical activity, which largely determines energy requirements, is difficult to estimate.

Physiology

Women have unique nutritional requirements, and in some cases need more nutrients than men; for example, women need twice as much calcium as men.

Pregnancy and Breastfeeding

During pregnancy and breastfeeding, women must ingest enough nutrients for themselves and their child, so they need significantly more protein and calories during these periods, as well as more vitamins and minerals (especially iron, iodine, calcium, folic acid, and vitamins A, C, and K). In 2001 the FAO of the UN reported that iron deficiency afflicted 43 percent of women in developing countries and increased the risk of death during childbirth. A 2008 review of interventions estimated that universal supplementation with calcium, iron, and folic acid during pregnancy could prevent 105,000 maternal deaths (23.6 percent of all maternal deaths).

Frequent pregnancies with short intervals between them and long periods of breastfeeding add an additional nutritional burden.

Educating Children

According to the FAO, women are often responsible for preparing food and have the chance to educate their children about beneficial food and health habits, giving mothers another chance to improve the nutrition of their children.

Elderly

Malnutrition and being underweight are more common in the elderly than in adults of other ages. If elderly people are healthy and active, the aging process alone does not usually cause malnutrition. However, changes in body composition, organ functions, adequate energy intake and ability to eat or access food are associated with aging, and may contribute to malnutrition. Sadness or depression can play a role, causing changes in appetite, digestion, energy level, weight, and well-being. A study on the relationship between malnutrition and other conditions in the elderly found that Malnutrition in the elderly can result from gastrointestinal and endocrine system disorders, loss of taste and smell, decreased appetite and inadequate dietary intake. Poor dental health, ill-fitting dentures, or chewing and swallowing problems can make eating difficult. As a result of these factors, malnutrition is seen to develop more easily in the elderly.

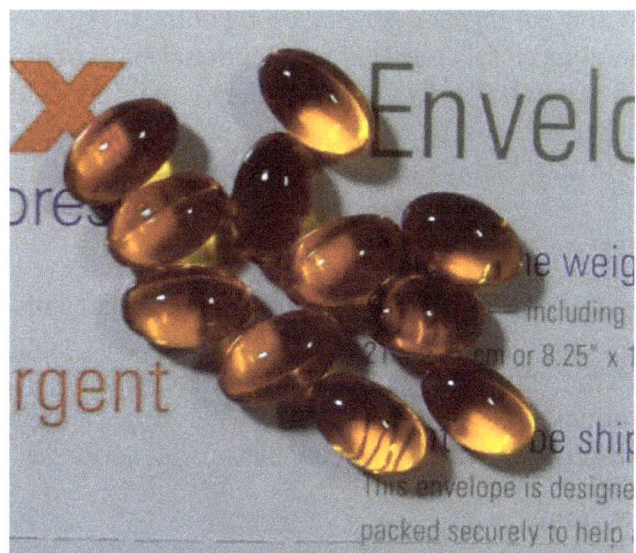

Essential nutrients are one of the main requirements of elderly care.

Rates of malnutrition tend to increase with age with less than 10 percent of the "young" elderly (up to age 75) malnourished, while 30 to 65 percent of the elderly in home care, long-term care facilities, or acute hospitals are malnourished. Many elderly people require assistance in eating, which may contribute to malnutrition. Because of this, one of the main requirements of elderly care is to provide an adequate diet and all essential nutrients.

In Australia malnutrition or risk of malnutrition occurs in 80 percent of elderly people presented to hospitals for admission. Malnutrition and weight loss can contribute to sarcopenia with loss of lean body mass and muscle function. Abdominal obesity or weight loss coupled with sarcopenia lead to immobility, skeletal disorders, insulin resistance, hypertension, atherosclerosis, and metabolic disorders. A paper from the *Journal of the American Dietetic Association* noted that routine nutrition screenings represent one way to detect and therefore decrease the prevalence of malnutrition in the elderly.

Pro-ana

Pro-ana refers to the promotion of behaviors related to the eating disorder anorexia nervosa. It is often referred to simply as ana. The lesser-used term pro-mia refers likewise to bulimia nervosa and is sometimes used interchangeably with pro-ana.

Pro-ana organizations differ widely in their stances. Most claim that they exist mainly as a non-judgmental environment for anorexics; a place to turn to, to discuss their illness, and to support those who choose to enter recovery. Others deny anorexia nervosa is a mental illness and claim instead that it is a "lifestyle choice" that should be respected by doctors and family.

The scientific community recognises anorexia nervosa as a serious illness. Some research suggests anorexia nervosa has the highest rate of mortality of any psychological disorder.

Culture

Medical professionals treating eating disorders have long noted that patients in recovery programs often "symptom pool", banding closely together for emotional support and validation. In this context, people with anorexia may collectively normalize their condition, defending it not as an illness but as an accomplishment of self-control and an essential part of their identity. Starving oneself becomes a lifestyle choice rather than an illness.

Online Presence

Such advocacy has flourished on the Internet, mainly through tight-knit support groups centred on web forums and, more recently, social network services such as Tumblr, Xanga, LiveJournal, Facebook and Myspace. These groups are typically small, vulnerable, partly hidden and characterized by frequent migrations. They also have an overwhelmingly female readership and are frequently the only means of support available to socially isolated anorexics.

Members of such support groups may:

- Endorse anorexia and/or bulimia as desirable (84% and 64% respectively in a 2010 survey).

- Share crash dieting techniques and recipes (67% of sites in a 2006 survey, rising to 83% in a 2010 survey).

- Coach each other on using socially acceptable pretexts for refusing food, such as veganism (which is notably more prevalent in the eating-disordered in general).

- Compete with each other at losing weight, or fast together in displays of solidarity.

- Commiserate with one another after breaking fast or binging.

- Advise on how to best induce vomiting, and on using laxatives and emetics.

- Give tips on hiding weight loss from parents and doctors.

- Share information on reducing the side-effects of anorexia.

- Post their weight, body measurements, details of their dietary regimen or pictures of themselves to solicit acceptance and affirmation.

- Suggest ways to ignore or suppress hunger pangs.

Many have popular blogs and forums on which members seek companionship by posting about their daily lives or boasting about personal accomplishments of weight loss. The communities centred on such sites can be warmly welcoming (especially in recovery-friendly groups) or sometimes cliquish and openly suspicious of newcomers. In particular, hostility is often leveled at:

- The non-eating disordered who express disapproval, including the spouses, relatives and friends of members who appear on-site to post threats and warnings.

- Casual dieters who join, believing that inducing eating disorders will cause them to lose weight more effectively. Such people are often derisively referred to as "wannabes" or "wannarexics".

Thinspiration

Pro-ana sites often (84%, in a 2010 survey) feature *thinspiration* (or *thinspo*): images or video montages of slim women, often celebrities, who may be anything from naturally slim to emaciated with visibly protruding bones. Pro-ana bloggers, forum members and social networking groups likewise post thinspiration to motivate one another toward further weight loss. Conversely, *reverse thinspiration* features images of fatty food or overweight people intended to induce disgust. There exists significant controversy between supporters and opponents of thinspiration; some assert that thinspiration only "glorifies" eating disorders while some thinspiration bloggers argue that the purpose of thinspiration is to support a healthy level of weight loss.

Thinspirational clips circulate widely on video sharing sites, pro-ana blogs often post thinspirational entries, and many pro-ana forums have threads dedicated to sharing thinspiration. Thinspiration can also take the form of inspirational mantras, quotes or selections of lyrics from poetry or popular music (94% of sites in a 2003 survey).

Thinspiration often has a spiritual-ascetic flavour, referring to fasting through metaphors of bodily purity, food through allusions to sin and corruption, and thinness through imagery of angels and angelic flight. Exhortations like "Ana's Creed" and "The Thin Commandments" are also common.

Appeal

Social researchers studying pro-ana have varied explanations for its popularity, with some characterizing it as a rejection of modern consumerism and others suggesting that pro-ana functions as a coping mechanism for those already emotionally stressed by eating disorders. Most, however, agree that pro-ana sites:

- Initially attract both the non-eating disordered (who first visit seeking tips and techniques for losing weight) and the eating-disordered (who seek advice on hiding their disordered behaviors, or minimizing the physical damage caused by over-exercising and severe calorie restriction).

- Give their members a strong sense of community and common identity.

Fashion

Red bracelets are popularly worn in pro-ana, both as a discreet way for anorexics to socially identify and as a tangible reminder to avoid eating. Pro-mia bracelets, likewise, are blue or purple. Most such bracelets are simple beaded items traded briskly on online auction sites.

Impact

Proliferation

Pro-ana has proliferated rapidly on the Internet, with some observers noting a first wave of pro-ana sites on free web hosting services in the late 1990s, and a second wave attributed to the recent rise of blogging and social networking services.

A survey by Internet security firm Optenet found a 470% increase in pro-ana and pro-mia sites from 2006 to 2007. A similar increase was also noted in a 2006 Maastricht University study investigating alternatives to censorship of pro-ana material. In the study, the Dutch blog host punt. nl began in October 2006 presenting visitors to pro-ana blogs on its service with a click-through warning containing a disparaging message and links to pro-recovery sites. Although the warnings were a deterrence (33.6% of the 530,000 unique visitors logged did not proceed past the warning), the number of such blogs actually increased tenfold, with their monthly traffic figures doubling on average by the end of the study.

Viewership

In a 2009 survey by the Katholieke Universiteit Leuven of 711 Flemish high school students aged 13–17, 12.6% of girls and 5.9% of boys reported having visited pro-ana websites at least once. In another 2009 survey, by parental control software vendor CyberSentinel of 1500 female Internet users aged 6–15, one in three reported having searched online for dieting tips, while one in five reported having corresponded with others on social networking sites or in chat rooms for tips on dieting.

Visitors to pro-ana web sites also include a significant number of those already diagnosed with eating disorders: a 2006 survey of eating disorder patients at Stanford Medical School found that 35.5% had visited pro-ana web sites; of those, 96.0% learned new weight loss or purging methods from such sites (while 46.4% of viewers of pro-recovery sites learned new techniques).

Effect

Pro-ana sites can negatively impact the eating behavior of people with and without eating disorders. One study of individuals without eating disorders demonstrated that 84% of participants decreased caloric intake by an average of 2,470 calories (301 min -7851 max) per week after viewing pro-ED (eating disorder) websites. Only 56% of participants actually perceived the reduction in their intake. Three weeks after the experiment, 24% of participants reported continuing weight control strategies from pro-ana websites, though they did not continue to visit those sites. Controls viewing health and travel websites did not decrease caloric intake at a significant level. Other studies have found that women with varying levels of eating disorder symptomatology were more likely to engage in image comparison and exercise after viewing pro-ana websites versus control websites.

Pro-ana sites can negatively impact cognition and affect. Women who viewed a pro-ana site, but not control sites focused on fashion or home décor, experienced an increase in negative affect and decreases in self-esteem, appearance self-efficacy, and perceived attractiveness. They also reported feeling heavier and being more likely to think about their weight. The effects of perfectionism, BMI, internalization of the thin ideal, and pre-existing ED symptomatology as moderators of negative affect were comparable to chance, suggesting that pro-ana websites can affect a broad spectrum of individuals, not simply those with ED characteristics.

A 2007 survey by the University of South Florida of 1575 girls and young women found that those who had a history of viewing pro-ana websites did not differ from those who viewed only pro-recovery websites on any of the survey's measures, including body mass index, negative body image, appearance dissatisfaction, level of disturbance, and dietary restriction. Those who had viewed pro-ana websites were, however, moderately more likely to have a negative body image than those who did not.

Similarly, girls in the 2009 Leuven survey who viewed pro-ana websites were more likely to have a negative body image and be dissatisfied with their body shape.

A 2012 report by Deloitte Access Economics, commissioned by Australian non-profit The Butterfly Foundation, estimated that eating disorders resulted in productivity losses totaling just over $AUD15 billion, with 1828 (515 males and 1313 females) dying that year from eating disorder-related complications.

Social Support vs. Exacerbation of Illness

Unlike pro-ana sites, pro-recovery sites are designed to encourage development and maintenance of healthy behaviors and cognitions. A study of pro-ana and pro-recovery website use among adolescents with eating disorders found that adolescents used both types of websites to further eating disordered behaviors. Those who viewed pro-ana sites were comparable to those who viewed pro-recovery sites with respect to appearance dissatisfaction, restriction, and bulimic behaviors. Over half of parents were unaware of any ED website usage.

People who use pro-ana sites report lower social support than controls and seek to fill this deficit by use of pro-ana sites. While pro-ana site users in this study perceived greater support from online communities than offline relationships, they also reported being encouraged to continue eating disorder behaviors. Users of pro-ana sites (n=60) cited a sense of belonging (77%), social support (75%), and support for the choice to continue current eating disorder behaviors (54%) as reasons for joining a pro-ana site. Reasons for continuing to use a pro-ana site included general support for stress (84%), meeting others with eating disorders (50%), and finding triggers for eating disorder behaviors (37%). Finally, behaviors first learned after visiting a pro-ana site include using thinspiration (63%), hiding eating disorder behaviors (60%), fasting (57%), using diuretics and laxatives (45%), vomiting (23%), using alcohol or other drugs to inhibit appetite (22%), and self-harm (22%).

Controversy and Criticism

Many medical professionals and some anorexics view pro-ana as a glamorization of a serious illness. Pro-ana began to attract attention from the mainstream press when *The Oprah Winfrey Show* aired a special episode in October 2001 focusing on pro-ana. Pressure from the public and pro-recovery organizations led to Yahoo and GeoCities shutting down pro-ana sites. In response, many groups now take steps to conceal themselves, disclaim their intentions as neutral and recovery-supportive (58% of sites in a 2006 survey), or interview members to screen out the non-eating disordered.

Medical Profession

Health care professionals and medical associations have generally negative views of pro-ana groups and the information they disseminate:

- The National Association of Anorexia Nervosa and Associated Disorders (ANAD) states that Pro-Ana sites "can pose a serious threat to some individuals, not simply because they promote eating disorder behaviors, but because they build a sense of community that is unhealthy. They lure the impressionable and persuade them that the Pro-Ana community is providing caring and nurturing advice."

- The Academy for Eating Disorders (AED) stated that "websites that glorify anorexia as a lifestyle choice play directly to the psychology of its victims", expressing concern that sites dedicated to the promotion of anorexia as a desirable "lifestyle choice" "provide support and encouragement to engage in health threatening behaviors, and neglect the serious consequences of starvation." However, one of its board members, Eric van Furth, has noted that pro-ana sites have relatively few visitors and advises against legal sanction of such sites, claiming instead that popular media play the more important role in establishing ideals of female thinness.

- Bodywhys (the Eating Disorders Association of Ireland) notes that pro-ana sites "might initially help people to feel less isolated, but the community that they create is an unhealthy community that encourages obsessiveness and minimization of the seriousness of these potentially deadly disorders."

- b-eat (the Eating Disorders Association of the UK) has remarked that those who seek out pro-ana sites do so "to find support, understanding and acceptance. We don't call for the sites to be banned, but rather for everyone else to consider how they can also provide that understanding and acceptance so that these sites don't become the only refuge for someone."

- The UK Royal College of Psychiatrists has called for the Council of Child Internet Safety—a UK government advisory body—to expand its definition of harmful online content to include pro-ana sites, and to inform parents and teachers of the dangers of pro-ana, arguing that "the broader societal context in which pro-ana and pro-mia sites thrive is one where young women are constantly bombarded with toxic images of supposed female perfection that are impossible to achieve, make women feel bad about themselves and significantly increase their risk of eating disorders."

- The National Eating Disorders Association (NEDA) "actively speaks out against pro-anorexia and pro-bulimia websites. These sites provide no useful information on treatment but instead encourage and falsely support those who, sadly, are ill but do not seek help." NEDA has also warned that journalists often glamorize anorexia by associating anorexia with personal self-control and that media coverage of pro-ana often triggers the already-anorexic by mentioning weights and calorie counts and by showing photographs of thin people.

Media

In October 2001, *The Oprah Winfrey Show* hosted a special on anorexia; the pro-ana movement was discussed briefly by the guest panel, who expressed alarm at the appearance of pro-ana websites and recommended the use of filtering software to bar access to them.

In July 2002, the *Baltimore City Paper* published an investigative report into pro-ana on the web.

"Growing up Online", a January 2008 episode of the PBS *Frontline* television program, also featured a brief discussion of pro-ana.

In April 2009, *The Truth about Online Anorexia*, an investigative documentary about pro-ana on the Internet, aired on ITV1 in the UK presented by BBC Radio 1 DJ Fearne Cotton.

In April 2012 speech at Harvard University, *Vogue Italia* editor Franca Sozzani conceded that the fashion industry may be a cause of the recent rise in eating disorders, but that the industry was being unfairly singled out for blame: "How can all this be possibly caused by fashion? And how come that Twiggy, who would be surely considered an anorexic today, did not arise controversy in the Sixties and did not produce a string of anorexia followers?" According to Sozzani, pro-ana sites were more effective at promoting eating disorders, and obesity was the more pressing public health problem that food industry was not being likewise attacked for exacerbating.

Arts

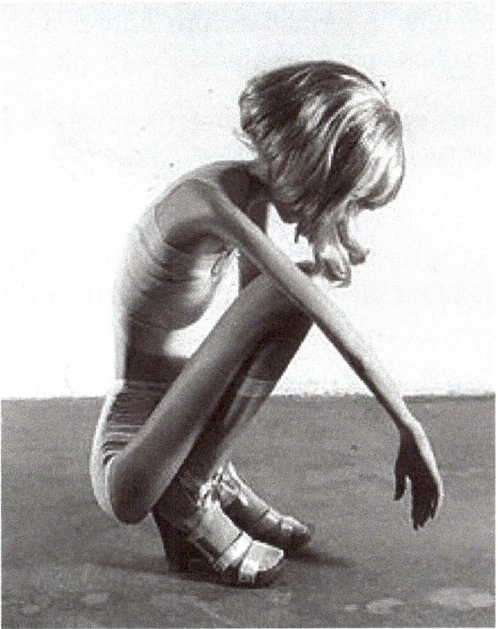

An image from Ivonne Thein's *Thirty-two kilos*,
a collection of digitally altered photographs satirizing thinspiration.

Thirty-two kilos, an exhibition by photographer Ivonne Thein, went on display at the Berlin Post-fuhramt art exhibition center in May 2008 and the Washington Goethe-Institut in January 2009, featuring photographs of young women digitally manipulated to appear skeletally thin. The photographs were intended as a mocking and satirical take on pro-ana. To Thein's dismay, however, many images from the exhibition were nevertheless later shared online as thinspiration.

Social Networking Services

In July 2001, Yahoo—after receiving a letter of complaint from ANAD—began removing pro-ana sites from its Yahoo Clubs (now Yahoo Groups) service, stating that such sites endorsing self-harm were violations of its terms of service agreement.

LiveJournal has not made a position statement on pro-ana. In August 2007, however, a staff member declined to act on an abuse report filed against a pro-ana community hosted on its network, stating that:

"Suspending pro-anorexia communities will not make anyone suffering from the disorder become healthy again. Allowing them to exist, however, has several benefits. It reassures those who join them that they are not alone in the way they feel about their bodies. It increases the chance that the friends and loved ones of the individuals in the community will discover their disorders and assist them in seeking professional help."

Facebook staff seek out and regularly delete pro-ana related groups. A spokesperson for the online service has stated that such pages violate the site's terms of service agreement by promoting self-harm in others.

MySpace does not ban pro-ana material and has stated that

"it's often very tricky to distinguish between support groups for users who are suffering from eating disorders and groups that might be termed as 'pro' anorexia or bulimia. Rather than censor these groups, we are working to create partnerships with organisations like b-eat."

MySpace has chosen instead to cycle banner advertisements for pro-recovery organizations through pro-ana members' profiles.

In November 2007, Microsoft shut down four pro-ana sites on the Spanish-language version of its Spaces social networking service at the behest of IQUA, the Internet regulatory body for Catalonia. A Microsoft spokesperson stated that such sites "infringe all the rules on content created by users and visible on our sites".

In September 2008, San Sebastián-based Spanish-language web portal Hispavista removed its pro-ana forums at the request of the provincial prosecutor for Guipúzcoa and the Children's Ombudsman of Madrid, who stated that "while not illegal, the harmful and false information in such forums being disseminated to minors will impair their proper development."

In February 2012, after consulting with NEDA, the blog-hosting service Tumblr announced that it would shut down blogs hosted on its microblogging service which "actively promote or glorify self harm," including eating disorders, and display warnings on searches for common pro-ana terms. Despite this, Tumblr remains a large hub for pro-ana microblogging. Pinterest, a social photo-sharing site, similarly amended its TOS in March 2012 to ban pro-ana content, but was similarly unsuccessful. Instagram followed suit and announced in April 2012 that it would summarily disable any accounts on its photo-sharing service with pro-ana specific hashtags on images.

Politics

In the United Kingdom, 40 MPs signed an early day motion tabled in February 2008 by the then Liberal Democrats member for Cheadle, Mark Hunter, urging government action against pro-ana sites. The motion was timed to coincide with the UK National Eating Disorder Awareness Week.

In the United Kingdom, Jo Swinson, the Liberal Democrat member for East Dunbartonshire, called for advertisers to voluntarily adopt similar disclaimers in an adjournment debate in October 2009, and later in an early day motion tabled in February 2010. She has stated that such "photos can lead people to believe in realities that, very often, do not exist," and that "when teenagers and women look at these pictures in magazines, they end up feeling unhappy with themselves."

In April 2008, a bill outlawing material which "provokes a person to seek excessive thinness by encouraging prolonged restriction of nourishment" was tabled in the French National Assembly by UMP MP Valérie Boyer. It imposes a fine of €30,000 and two years imprisonment (rising to €45,000 and three years if there was a resulting death) on offenders. Health minister Roselyne Bachelot, arguing for the bill, stated that "giving young girls advice about how to lie to their doctors, telling them what kinds of food are easiest to vomit, encouraging them to torture themselves whenever they take any kind of food is not part of liberty of expression." The bill passed the National Assembly, but stalled in the Senate, where a June 2008 report by the Committee of Social Affairs emphatically recommended against such legislation and instead suggested early-screening programs by schools and physicians.

Boyer subsequently introduced another bill in September 2009 to mandate disclaimers on photographs in which body parts have been retouched, with the aim of reducing the impact of unrealism in photography on young girls and women. The bill was ostensibly targeted at advertising photography but could be broadly applicable to digitally manipulated photography in general, including thinspirational montages. It imposes a penalty of €37,500 per violation, with a possible rise to 50% of the cost of each advertisement. The bill did not pass its first reading and was relegated to the Committee of Social Affairs.

In April 2009, Dutch Minister for Youth and Family André Rouvoet called for click-through warnings to be added to all pro-ana sites on Dutch hosting services, citing a successful trial of such warnings by blog host punt.nl in 2006. The Dutch Hosting Provider Association, however, has stated that "the Internet is simply a reflection of a world with many undesirable things", and that its members cannot be held responsible for monitoring and disclaiming all hosted content.

In March 2012, the Israeli Knesset passed a bill sponsored by Kadima MK Rachel Adato and Likud MK Danny Danon requiring advertisements which have been retouched to alter the body shape of models to fully disclose the fact. The bill, which applies to both foreign-produced and locally produced advertising, also sets a lower BMI limit for models featured in advertisements of 18.5 (the threshold of underweight under World Health Organization guidelines).

Popular Culture

In a November 2009 interview with *Women's Wear Daily*, model Kate Moss gave a popular thin-spirational slogan as her motto: "Nothing tastes as good as skinny feels." Moss came under wide-spread criticism—particularly by eating disorder recovery organizations—for endorsing pro-ana. Her agency, Storm, stated: "This was part of a longer answer Kate gave during a wider ranging interview which has unfortunately been taken out of context and misrepresented." Still, Moss has been known in the fashion world to have helped popularize the "heroin chic" trend, which uses models with disheveled, ultra-skinny, and waif-like body types on the runway.

Hypergymnasia

Anorexia athletica (sports anorexia), also referred to as hypergymnasia is an eating disorder char-acterized by excessive and compulsive exercise. An athlete suffering from sports anorexia tends to over exercise to give themselves a sense of having control over their body. Most often, people with the disorder tend to feel they have no control over their lives other than their control of food and exercise. In actuality, they have no control; they cannot stop exercising or regulating food intake without feeling guilty. Generally, once the activity is started, it is difficult to stop because the per-son is seen as being addicted to the method adopted.

Anorexia athletica is used to refer to "a disorder for athletes who engage in at least one unhealthy method of weight control". Unlike anorexia nervosa, anorexia athletica does not have as much to do with body image as it does with performance. Athletes usually begin by eating more 'healthy' foods, as well as increasing their training, but when people feel like that is not enough and start working out excessively and cutting back their caloric intake until it becomes a psychological dis-order.

Hypergymnasia and anorexia athletica are not recognized as mental disorders in any of the med-ical manuals, such as the ICD-10 or the DSM-IV, nor is it part of the proposed revision of this manual, the DSM-5. If this were the case, there would be a 10–15% increase in mental disorders in sports. A study at the Anorexia Centre at Huddinge Hospital in Stockholm, Sweden showed that sports anorexia can result in mental disorders. The anxiety, stress, and pressure people with sports anorexia put on themselves (as well as the pressure parents and coaches can put on the athlete) can cause mental disorders.

Signs and Symptoms

Someone with anorexia athletica can experience numerous signs and symptoms, a few of which are listed below. The seriousness of the symptoms is dependent on the individual, and more symp-toms come with the length the athlete excessively exercises. If anorexia athletica persists for long enough, the individual can become malnourished, which eventually leads to further complications in major organs such as the liver, kidney, heart and brain.

- Excessive exercise

- Obsessive behaviour with calories, fat, and weight

- Self-worth is based on physical performance

- Enjoyment of sports is diminished or gone

- Denying the over exercising is a problem

Causes

There is not one single cause of anorexia athletica, but many factors that are involved in the disorder. Research has shown that an area on chromosome 1 is linked to anorexia nervosa-sports anorexia. Thus, a person is more likely to have anorexia athletica if someone in their immediate family has had the disorder. Not only genetics, but also the environment a person is in, has a major impact on the disorder. Coaches and parents often suggest to their athlete/child to lose weight in order to perform better. Sports such as figure skating, ballet, and gymnastics promote both male and female athletes to have a thin figure. Females who partake in sports can suffer from a syndrome known as the triad. The media play a very significant role in pressuring athletes to have the 'perfect' body and to be thin, which can also trigger sports anorexia.

Treatment

According to the National Eating Disorder Information Centre (NEDIC), the first step for someone going through anorexia athletica is to realize their eating and exercise habits are hurting them. Once an individual has realized they have a disorder, an appointment should be made with the family doctor. A family doctor can advise further medical attention if needed. With sports anorexia, it is important to go to a dietitian as well as a personal trainer. People with sports anorexia need to learn the balance between exercise and caloric intake.

Bulimia Nervosa

Bulimia nervosa, also known as simply bulimia, is an eating disorder characterized by binge eating followed by purging. Binge eating refers to eating a large amount of food in a short amount of time. Purging refers to the attempts to get rid of the food consumed. This may be done by vomiting or taking laxatives. Other efforts to lose weight may include the use of diuretics, stimulants, water fasting, or excessive exercise. Most people with bulimia are at a normal weight. The forcing of vomiting may result in thickened skin on the knuckles and breakdown of the teeth. Bulimia is frequently associated with other mental disorders such as depression, anxiety, and problems with drugs or alcohol. There is also a higher risk of suicide and self-harm.

Bulimia is more common among those who have a close relative with the condition. The percentage risk that is estimated to be due to genetics is between 30% and 80%. Other risk factors for the disease include psychological stress, cultural pressure to attain a certain body type, poor self-esteem, and obesity. Living in a culture that promotes dieting and having parents that worry about weight are also risks. Diagnosis is based on a person's medical history, however this is difficult as people are usually secretive about their binge eating and purging habits. Furthermore, the diagnosis of anorexia nervosa takes precedence over that of bulimia. Other similar disorders include binge eating disorder, Kleine-Levin syndrome, and borderline personality disorder.

Cognitive behavioral therapy is the primary treatment for bulimia. Antidepressants of the selective serotonin reuptake inhibitors (SSRI) or tricyclic antidepressant class may have a modest benefit. While outcomes with bulimia are typically better than in those of anorexia, the risk of death among those affected is higher than that of the general population. At 10 years after receiving treatment about 50% of people are fully recovered.

Globally, bulimia was estimated to affect 3.6 million people in 2015. About 1% of young women have bulimia at a given point in time and about 2% to 3% of women have the condition at some point in their lives. The condition is less common in the developing world. Bulimia is about nine times more likely to occur in women than men. Among women, rates are highest in young adults. Bulimia was named and first described by the British psychiatrist Gerald Russell in 1979.

Signs and Symptoms

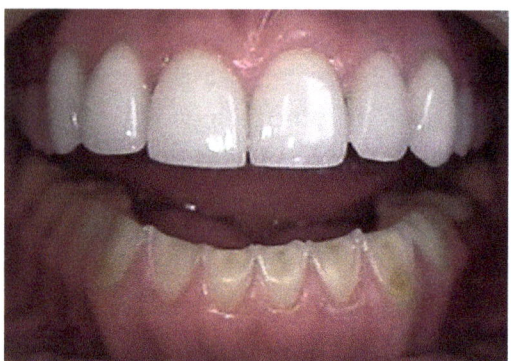

The erosion on the lower teeth was caused by bulimia. For comparison, the upper teeth were restored with porcelain veneers.

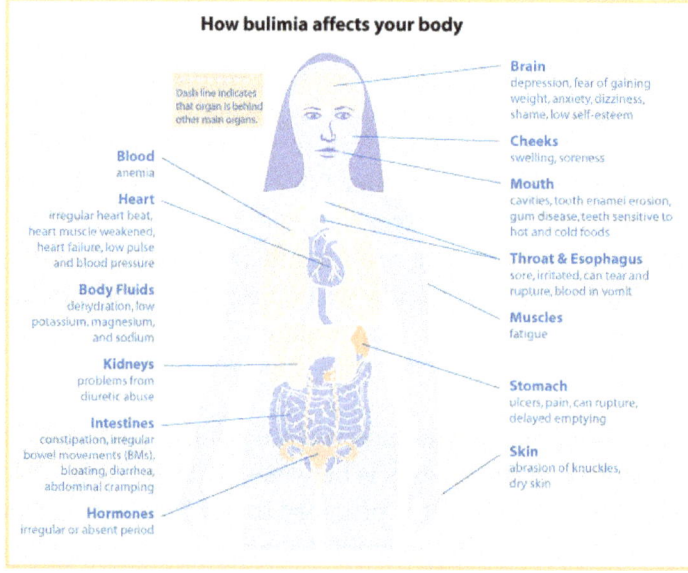

How bulimia affects the body

Bulimia typically involves rapid and out-of-control eating, which may stop when the bulimic is interrupted by another person or the stomach hurts from over-extension, followed by self-induced vomiting or other forms of purging. This cycle may be repeated several times a week or, in more serious cases, several times a day and may directly cause:

- Chronic gastric reflux after eating, secondary to vomiting

- Dehydration and hypokalemia due to renal potassium loss in the presence of alkalosis and frequent vomiting

- Electrolyte imbalance, which can lead to abnormal heart rhythms, cardiac arrest, and even death

- Esophagitis, or inflammation of the esophagus

- Mallory-Weiss tears

- Boerhaave syndrome, a rupture in the esophageal wall due to vomiting

- Oral trauma, in which repetitive insertion of fingers or other objects causes lacerations to the lining of the mouth or throat

- Russell's sign: calluses on knuckles and back of hands due to repeated trauma from incisors

- Perimolysis, or severe dental erosion of tooth enamel

- Swollen salivary glands (for example, in the neck, under the jaw line)

- Gastroparesis or delayed emptying

- Constipation

- Peptic ulcers

- Infertility

- Constant weight fluctuations are common

These are some of the many signs that may indicate whether someone has bulimia nervosa:

- A fixation on the number of calories consumed.

- A fixation on and extreme consciousness of ones weight.

- Low self-esteem and/or self harming.

- Suicidal tendencies

- Low blood pressure

- An irregular menstrual cycle in woman.

- Regular trips to the bathroom, especially soon after eating.

- Depression, anxiety disorders and sleep disorders.

- Frequent occurrences involving consumption of abnormally large portions of food.

- The use of laxatives and diet pills.

- Unhealthy/dry skin, hair, nails and lips.

- A lack of energy.

As with many psychiatric illnesses, delusions can occur, in conjunction with other signs and symptoms, leaving the person with a false belief that is not ordinarily accepted by others.

People with bulimia nervosa may also exercise to a point that excludes other activities.

Related Disorders

Bulimics are much more likely than non-bulimics to have an affective disorder, such as depression or general anxiety disorder: A 1985 Columbia University study on female bulimics at New York State Psychiatric Institute found 70% had suffered depression some time in their lives (as opposed to 25.8% for adult females in a control sample from the general population), rising to 88% for all affective disorders combined. Another study by the Royal Children's Hospital in Melbourne on a cohort of 2,000 adolescents similarly found that those meeting at least two of the DSM-IV criteria for bulimia nervosa or anorexia nervosa had a sixfold increase in risk of anxiety and a doubled risk for substance dependency. Some sufferers of anorexia nervosa exhibit episodes of bulimic tendencies through purging (either through self-induced vomiting or laxatives) as a way to quickly remove food in their system. Bulimia also has negative effects on the sufferer's dental health due to the acid passed through the mouth from frequent vomiting causing acid erosion, mainly on the posterior dental surface.

Diagnosis

The onset of bulimia nervosa is often during adolescence, between 13 and 20 years of age, and many cases have previously suffered from obesity, with many sufferers relapsing in adulthood into episodic bingeing and purging even after initially successful treatment and remission. A lifetime prevalence of 0.5 percent and 0.9 percent for adult and adolescent sufferers, respectively, is estimated among the United States population. Bulimia nervosa may affect up to 1% of young women and, after 10 years of diagnosis, half will recover fully, a third will recover partially, and 10–20% will still have symptoms.

Adolescents with bulimia nervosa are more likely to have self-imposed perfectionism and compulsivity issues in eating compared to their peers. This means that the high expectations and unrealistic goals that these individuals set for themselves are internally motivated rather than by social views or expectations.

Criteria

Bulimia nervosa can be difficult to detect, compared to anorexia nervosa, because bulimics tend to be of average or slightly above or below average weight. Many bulimics may also engage in significantly disordered eating and exercise patterns without meeting the full diagnostic criteria for bulimia nervosa. Recently, the *Diagnostic and Statistical Manual of Mental Disorders* was revised, which resulted in the loosening of criteria regarding the diagnoses of bulimia nervosa and anorexia nervosa. The diagnostic criteria utilized by the DSM-5 includes repetitive episodes of binge eating (a discrete episode of overeating during which the individual feels out of control of consumption) compensated for by excessive or inappropriate measures taken to avoid gaining weight. The diagnosis also requires the episodes of compensatory behaviors and binge eating to happen a minimum of once a week for a consistent time period of 3 months. The diagnosis is made only when the behavior is not a part of the symptom complex of anorexia nervosa and when the behavior reflects an overemphasis on physical mass or appearance. Purging often is a common characteristic of a more severe case of bulimia nervosa.

Causes

Biological

As with anorexia nervosa, there is evidence of genetic predispositions contributing to the onset of this eating disorder. Abnormal levels of many hormones, notably serotonin, have been shown to be responsible for some disordered eating behaviors. Brain-derived neurotrophic factor (BDNF) is under investigation as a possible mechanism.

There is evidence that sex hormones may influence appetite and eating in women, and the onset of bulimia nervosa. Studies have shown that women with hyperandrogenism and polycystic ovary syndrome have a dysregulation of appetite, along with carbohydrates and fats. This dysregulation of appetite is also seen in women with bulimia nervosa. In addition, gene knockout studies in mice have shown that mice that have the gene encoding estrogen receptors have decreased fertility due to ovarian dysfunction and dysregulation of androgen receptors. In humans, there is evidence that there is an association between polymorphisms in the ERβ (estrogen receptor β) and bulimia, suggesting there is a correlation between sex hormones and bulimia nervosa.

Bulimia has been compared to drug addiction, though the empirical support for this characterization is limited. However, people with bulimia nervosa may share dopamine D2 receptor-related vulnerabilities with those with substance abuse disorders.

Dieting, a common behaviour in bulimics, is associated with lower plasma tryptophan levels. Decreased tryptophan levels in the brain, and thus the synthesis of serotonin, increases bulimic urges in currently and formerly bulimic individuals within hours.

Social

Media portrayals of an 'ideal' body shape are widely considered to be a contributing factor to bulimia. In a 1991 study by Weltzin, Hsu, Pollicle, and Kaye, it was stated that 19% of bulimics undereat, 37% of bulimics eat an amount of food that is normal for an average human being, and 44% of bulimics overeat. A survey of 15- to 18-year-old high school girls in Nadroga, Fiji, found the self-reported incidence of purging rose from 0% in 1995 (a few weeks after the introduction of television in the province) to 11.3% in 1998. In addition, the suicide rate among people with bulimia nervosa is 7.5 times higher than in the general population.

When attempting to decipher the origin of bulimia nervosa in a cognitive context, Christopher Fairburn *et al.*'s cognitive behavioral model is often considered the golden standard. Fairburn et al.'s model discusses the process in which an individual falls into the binge-purge cycle and thus develops bulimia. Fairburn *et al.* argue that extreme concern with weight and shape coupled with low self-esteem will result in strict, rigid, and inflexible dietary rules. Accordingly, this would lead to unrealistically restricted eating, which may consequently induce an eventual "slip" where the individual commits a minor infraction of the strict and inflexible dietary rules. Moreover, the cognitive distortion due to dichotomous thinking leads the individual to binge. The binge subsequently should trigger a perceived loss of control, promoting the individual to purge in hope of counteracting the binge. However, Fairburn *et al.* assert the cycle repeats itself, and thus consider the binge-purge cycle to be self-perpetuating.

In contrast, Byrne and Mclean's findings differed slightly from Fairburn *et al.*'s cognitive behavioral model of bulimia nervosa in that the drive for thinness was the major cause of purging as a way of controlling weight. In turn, Byrne and Mclean argued that this makes the individual vulnerable to binging, indicating that it is not a binge-purge cycle but rather a purge-binge cycle in that purging comes before bingeing. Similarly, Fairburn *et al.*'s cognitive behavioral model of bulimia nervosa is not necessarily applicable to every individual and is certainly reductionist. Everyone differs from another, and taking such a complex behavior like bulimia and applying the same one theory to everyone would certainly be invalid. In addition, the cognitive behavioral model of bulimia nervosa is very cultural bound in that it may not be necessarily applicable to cultures outside of the Western society. To evaluate, Fairburn *et al.*.'s model and more generally the cognitive explanation of bulimia nervosa is more descriptive than explanatory, as it does not necessarily explain how bulimia arises. Furthermore, it is difficult to ascertain cause and effect, because it may be that distorted eating leads to distorted cognition rather than vice versa.

A considerable amount of literature has identified a correlation between sexual abuse and the development of bulimia nervosa. The reported incident rate of unwanted sexual contact is higher among those with bulimia nervosa than anorexia nervosa.

When exploring the etiology of bulimia through a socio-cultural perspective, the "thin ideal internalization" is significantly responsible. The thin ideal internalization is the extent to which individuals adapt to the societal ideals of attractiveness. Studies have shown that young females that read fashion magazines tend to have more bulimic symptoms than those females who do not. This further demonstrates the impact of media on the likelihood of developing the disorder. Individuals first accept and "buy into" the ideals, and then attempt to transform themselves in order to reflect the societal ideals of attractiveness. J. Kevin Thompson and Eric Stice claim that family, peers, and most evidently media reinforce the thin ideal, which may lead to an individual accepting and "buying into" the thin ideal. In turn, Thompson and Stice assert that if the thin ideal is accepted, one could begin to feel uncomfortable with their body shape or size since it may not necessarily reflect the thin ideal set out by society. Thus, people feeling uncomfortable with their bodies may result in suffering from body dissatisfaction and may develop a certain drive for thinness. Consequently, body dissatisfaction coupled with a drive for thinness is thought to promote dieting and negative effects, which could eventually lead to bulimic symptoms such as purging or bingeing. Binges lead to self-disgust which causes purging to prevent weight gain.

A study dedicated to investigating the thin ideal internalization as a factor of bulimia nervosa is Thompson's and Stice's research. The aim of their study was to investigate how and to what degree does media affect the thin ideal internalization. Thompson and Stice used randomized experiments (more specifically programs) dedicated to teaching young women how to be more critical when it comes to media, in order to reduce thin ideal internalization. The results showed that by creating more awareness of the media's control of the societal ideal of attractiveness, the thin ideal internalization significantly dropped. In other words, less thin ideal images portrayed by the media resulted in less thin ideal internalization. Therefore, Thompson and Stice concluded that media affected greatly the thin ideal internalization. Papies showed that it is not the thin ideal itself, but rather the self-association with other persons of a certain weight that decide how someone with bulimia nervosa feels. People that associate themselves with thin models get in a positive attitude when they see thin models and people that associate with overweight get in a negative attitude when they see thin models. Moreover, it can be taught to associate with thinner people.

Treatment

There are two main types of treatment given to those suffering with bulimia nervosa; psychopharmacological and psychosocial treatments.

Psychotherapy

There are several supported psychosocial treatments for bulimia. Cognitive behavioral therapy (CBT), which involves teaching a person to challenge automatic thoughts and engage in behavioral experiments (for example, in session eating of "forbidden foods") has a small amount of evidence supporting its use.

By using CBT people record how much food they eat and periods of vomiting with the purpose of identifying and avoiding emotional fluctuations that bring on episodes of bulimia on a regular basis. Barker (2003) states that research has found 40–60% of people using cognitive behaviour therapy to become symptom free. He states in order for the therapy to work, all parties must work together to discuss, record and develop coping strategies. Barker (2003) claims by making people aware of their actions they will think of alternatives. People undergoing CBT who exhibit early behavioral changes are most likely to achieve the best treatment outcomes in the long run. Researchers have also reported some positive outcomes for interpersonal psychotherapy and dialectical behavior therapy.

Maudsley family therapy, developed at the Maudsley Hospital in London for the treatment of anorexia has been shown promising results in bulimia.

The use of Cognitive Behavioral Therapy (CBT) has been shown to be quite effective for treating bulimia nervosa (BN) in adults, but little research has been done on effective treatments of BN for adolescents. Although CBT is seen as more cost efficient and helps individuals with BN in self-guided care, Family Based Treatment (FBT) might be more helpful to younger adolescents who need more support and guidance from their families. Adolescents are at the stage where their brains are still quite malleable and developing gradually. Therefore, young adolescents with BN are less likely to realize the detrimental consequences of becoming bulimic and have less motivation to change, which is why FBT would be useful to have families intervene and support the teens. Working with BN patients and their families in FBT can empower the families by having them involved in their adolescent's food choices and behaviors, taking more control of the situation in the beginning and gradually letting the adolescent become more autonomous when they have learned healthier eating habits.

Medication

Antidepressants of the selective serotonin reuptake inhibitors (SSRI) class may have a modest benefit. This includes fluoxetine, which is FDA approved, for the treatment of bulimia, other antidepressants such as sertraline may also be effective against bulimia. Topiramate may also be useful but has greater side effects.

It is not known if combining medication with counseling improves the outcomes. Any trials which originally suggested that such combinations should improve the outcome have not proven to be exceptionally powerful. Some positive outcomes of treatments can include: abstinence from binge eating, a decrease in obsessive behaviors to lose weight and in shape preoccupation, less severe psychiatric symptoms, a desire to counter the effects of binge eating, as well as an improvement in social functioning and reduced relapse rates.

Alternative Medicine

Some researchers have also claimed positive outcomes in hypnotherapy.

Epidemiology

There is little data on the percentage of people with bulimia in general populations. Most studies conducted thus far have been on convenience samples from hospital patients, high school or university students. These have yielded a wide range of results: between 0.1% and 1.4% of males, and between 0.3% and 9.4% of females. Studies on time trends in the prevalence of bulimia nervosa have also yielded inconsistent results. According to Gelder, Mayou and Geddes (2005) bulimia nervosa is prevalent between 1 and 2 percent of women aged 15–40 years. Bulimia nervosa occurs more frequently in developed countries and in cities, with one study finding that bulimia is five times more prevalent in cities than in rural areas. There is a perception that bulimia is most prevalent amongst girls from middle-class families; however, in a 2009 study girls from families in the lowest income bracket studied were 153 percent more likely to be bulimic than girls from the highest income bracket.

There are higher rates of eating disorders in groups involved in activities which idealize a slim physique, such as dance, gymnastics, modeling, cheerleading, running, acting, swimming, diving, rowing and figure skating. Bulimia is thought to be more prevalent among Caucasians; however, a more recent study showed that African-American teenage girls were 50 percent more likely than white girls to exhibit bulimic behavior, including both binging and purging.

Country	Year	Sample size and type	% affected	
Australia	2008	1,943 adolescents (ages 15–17)	1.0% male	6.4% female
Portugal	2006	2,028 high school students		0.3% female
Brazil	2004	1,807 students (ages 7–19)	0.8% male	1.3% female
Spain	2004	2,509 female adolescents (ages 13–22)		1.4% female
Hungary	2003	580 Budapest residents	0.4% male	3.6% female
Australia	1998	4,200 high school students	0.3% combined	

United States	1996	1,152 college students	0.2% male	1.3% female
Norway	1995	19,067 psychiatric patients	0.7% male	7.3% female
Canada	1995	8,116 (random sample)	0.1% male	1.1% female
Japan	1995	2,597 high school students	0.7% male	1.9% female
United States	1992	799 college students	0.4% male	5.1% female

History

Etymology

The term *bulimia* comes from Greek *boulīmia*, "ravenous hunger", a compound of *bous*, "ox" and *līmos*, "hunger". Literally, the scientific name of the disorder, *bulimia nervosa*, translates to "nervous ravenous hunger".

Before the 20th Century

Although diagnostic criteria for bulimia nervosa did not appear until 1979, evidence suggests that binging and purging were popular in certain ancient cultures. The first documented account of behavior resembling bulimia nervosa was recorded in Xenophon's Anabasis around 370 B.C, in which Greek soldiers purged themselves in the mountains of Asia Minor. It is unclear whether this purging was preceded by binging. In ancient Egypt, physicians recommended purging once a month for three days in order to preserve health. This practice stemmed from the belief that human diseases were caused by the food itself. In ancient Rome, elite society members would vomit in order to "make room" in their stomachs for more food at all day banquets. Emperors Claudius and Vitellius both were gluttonous and obese, and they often resorted to habitual purging.

Historical records also suggest that some saints who developed anorexia (as a result of a life of asceticism) may also have displayed bulimic behaviors. Saint Mary Magdalen de Pazzi (1566–1607) and Saint Veronica Giuliani (1660–1727) were both observed binge eating—giving in, as they believed, to the temptations of the devil. Saint Catherine of Siena (1347–1380) is known to have supplemented her strict abstinence from food by purging as reparation for her sins. Catherine died from starvation at age thirty-three.

While the psychological disorder "bulimia nervosa" is relatively new, the word "bulimia," signifying overeating, has been present for centuries. The Babylon Talmud referenced practices of "bulimia," yet scholars believe that this simply referred to overeating without the purging or the psychological implications bulimia nervosa. In fact, a search for evidence of bulimia nervosa from the 17th to late 19th century revealed that only a quarter of the overeating cases they examined actually vomited after the binges. There was no evidence of deliberate vomiting or an attempt to control weight.

20th Century

At the turn of the century, bulimia (overeating) was described as a clinical symptom, but rarely in the context of weight control. Purging, however, was seen in anorexic patients and attributed to gastric pain rather than another method of weight control.

In 1930, admissions of anorexia nervosa patients to the Mayo Clinic from 1917 to 1929 were compiled. Fifty-five to sixty-five percent of these patients were reported to be voluntarily vomiting in order to relieve weight anxiety. Records show that purging for weight control continued throughout the mid-1900s. Several case studies from this era reveal patients suffering from the modern description of bulimia nervosa. In 1939, Rahman and Richardson reported that out of their six anorexic patients, one had periods of overeating and another practiced self-induced vomiting. Wulff, in 1932, treated "Patient D," who would have periods of intense cravings for food and overeat for weeks, which often resulted in frequent vomiting. Patient D, who grew up with a tyrannical father, was repulsed by her weight and would fast for a few days, rapidly losing weight. Ellen West, a patient described by Ludwig Binswanger in 1958, was teased by friends for being fat and excessively took thyroid pills to lose weight, later using laxatives and vomiting. She reportedly consumed dozens of oranges and several pounds of tomatoes each day, yet would skip meals. After being admitted to a psychiatric facility for depression, Ellen ate ravenously yet lost weight, presumably due to self-induced vomiting. However, while these patients may have met modern criteria for bulimia nervosa, they cannot technically be diagnosed with the disorder, as it had not yet appeared in the Diagnostic and Statistical Manual of Mental Disorders at the time of their treatment.

An explanation for the increased instances of bulimic symptoms may be due to the 20th century's new ideals of thinness. The shame of being fat emerged in the 1940s, when teasing remarks about weight became more common. The 1950s, however, truly introduced the trend of an aspiration for thinness.

In 1979, Gerald Russell first published a description of bulimia nervosa, in which he studied patients with a "morbid fear of becoming fat" who overate and purged afterwards. He specified treatment options and indicated the seriousness of the disease, which can be accompanied by depression and suicide. In 1980, bulimia nervosa first appeared in the DSM-III.

After its appearance in the DSM-III, there was a sudden rise in the documented incidences of bulimia nervosa. In the early 1980s, incidences of the disorder rose to about 40 in every 100,000 people. This decreased to about 27 in every 100,000 people at the end of the 1980s/early 1990s. However, bulimia nervosa's prevalence was still much higher than anorexia nervosa's, which at the time occurred in about 14 people per 100,000.

In 1991, Kendler et al. documented the cumulative risk for bulimia nervosa for those born before 1950, from 1950 to 1959, and after 1959. The risk for those born after 1959 is much higher than those in either of the other cohorts.

Binge Eating Disorder

Binge eating disorder (BED) is an eating disorder characterized by frequent and recurrent binge eating episodes with associated negative psychological and social problems, but without subsequent purging episodes (e.g. vomiting).

BED is a recently described condition, which was required to distinguish binge eating similar to that seen bulimia nervosa but without characteristic purging. Individuals who are diagnosed with bulimia nervosa and binge eating disorder exhibit similar patterns of compulsive overeating, neurobiological features of dysfunctional cognitive control and food addiction, and biological and environmental risk factors. Indeed, some consider BED a milder version of bulimia nervosa, and that the conditions are on the same spectrum.

Binge eating is one of the most prevalent eating disorders among adults, though there tends to be less media coverage and research about the disorder in comparison to anorexia nervosa and bulimia nervosa.

Signs and Symptoms

Binge eating is the core symptom of BED; however, not everyone who binge eats has BED. An individual may occasionally binge eat without experiencing many of the negative physical, psychological, or social effects of BED. This example may be considered an eating problem (or not), rather than a disorder. Precisely defining binge eating can be problematic, however binge eating episodes in BED are generally described as having the following potential features:

- Eating much faster than normal during a binge perhaps in a short space of time

- Eating until feeling uncomfortably full

- Eating a large amount when not hungry

- Subjective loss of control over how much or what is eaten

- Binges may be planned in advance, involving the purchase of special binge foods, and the allocation of specific time for binging, sometimes at night

- Eating alone or secretly due to embarrassment over the amount of food consumed

- There may be a dazed mental state during the binge

- Not being able to remember what was eaten after the binge

- Feelings of guilt, shame or disgust following a food binge

In contrast to bulimia nervosa, binge eating episodes are not regularly followed by activities intended to prevent weight gain, such as self-induced vomiting, laxative or enema misuse, or strenuous exercise. BED is characterized more by overeating than dietary restriction and over concern about body shape. Obesity is common in persons with BED, as are depressive features, low self-esteem, stress and boredom.

Causes

As with other eating disorders, binge eating is an "expressive disorder"—a disorder that is an expression of deeper psychological problems. People who suffer from binge eating disorder have been found to have higher weight bias internalization, which includes low self-esteem, unhealthy eating patterns, and general body dissatisfaction. Binge eating disorder commonly develops as a result or side effect of depression, as it is common for people to turn to comfort foods when they are feeling down.

There was resistance to give binge eating disorder the status of a fully fledged eating disorder because many perceived binge eating disorder to be caused by individual choices. Previous research has focused on the relationship between body image and eating disorders, and concludes that disordered eating might be linked to rigid dieting practices. In the majority of cases of anorexia, extreme and inflexible restriction of dietary intake leads at some point to the development of binge eating, weight regain, bulimia nervosa, or a mixed form of eating disorder not otherwise specified. Binge eating may begin when individuals recover from an adoption of rigid eating habits. When under a strict diet that mimics the effects of starvation, the body may be preparing for a new type of behavior pattern, one that consumes a large amount of food in a relatively short period of time.

However, other research suggests that binge eating disorder can also be caused by environmental factors and the impact of traumatic events. One study showed that women with binge eating disorder experienced more adverse life events in the year prior to the onset of the development of the disorder, and that binge eating disorder was positively associated with how frequently negative events occur. Additionally, the research found that individuals who had binge eating disorder were more likely to have experienced physical abuse, perceived risk of physical abuse, stress, and body criticism. Other risk factors may include childhood obesity, critical comments about weight, low self-esteem, depression, and physical or sexual abuse in childhood. A few studies have suggested that there could be a genetic component to binge eating disorder, though other studies have shown more ambiguous results. Studies have shown that binge eating tends to run in families and a twin study by Bulik, Sullivan, and Kendler has shown a, "moderate heritability for binge eating" at 41 percent. More research must be done before any firm conclusions can be drawn regarding the heritability of binge eating disorder. Studies have also shown that eating disorders such as anorexia and bulimia reduce coping abilities, which makes it more likely for those suffering to turn to binge eating as a coping strategy.

A correlation between dietary restraint and the occurrence of binge eating has been shown in some research. While binge eaters are often believed to be lacking in self-control, the root of such behavior might instead be linked to rigid dieting practices. The relationship between strict dieting and binge eating is characterized by a vicious circle. Binge eating is more likely to occur after dieting, and vice versa. Several forms of dieting include delay in eating (e.g., not eating during the day), restriction of overall calorie intake (e.g., setting calorie limit to 1,000 calories per day), and avoidance of certain types of food (e.g., "forbidden" food, such as sugar, carbohydrates, etc.) Strict and extreme dieting differs from ordinary dieting. Some evidence suggests the effectiveness of moderate calorie restriction in decreasing binge eating episodes among overweight individuals with binge eating disorder, at least in the short-term.

Diagnosis

International Statistical Classification of Diseases and Related Health Problems

The 2017 update to the American version of the ICD-10 includes BED under F50.81. ICD-11 may contain a dedicated entry (6B62), defining BED as frequent, recurrent episodes of binge eating (once a week or more over a period of several months) which are not regularly followed by inappropriate compensatory behaviors aimed at preventing weight gain.

Diagnostic and Statistical Manual of Mental Disorders

Previously considered a topic for further research exploration, binge eating disorder was included in the *Diagnostic and Statistical Manual of Mental Disorders* in 2013. Until 2013, binge eating disorder was categorized as an Eating Disorder Not Otherwise Specified, an umbrella category for eating disorders that don't fall under the categories for anorexia nervosa or bulimia nervosa. Because it was not a recognized psychiatric disorder in the *DSM-IV* until 2013, it has been difficult to obtain insurance reimbursement for treatments. The disorder now has its own category under *DSM-5*, which outlines the signs and symptoms that must be present to classify a person's behavior as binge eating disorder. Studies have confirmed the high predictive value of these criteria for diagnosing BED.

According to DSM-5, the following criteria must be present to make a diagnosis of binge eating disorder. Studies have confirmed the high predictive value of these criteria for diagnosing BED. A. Recurrent episodes of binge eating. An episode of binge eating is characterized by both of the following:

1. Eating, in a discrete period of time (e.g., within any 2-hour period), an amount of food that is definitely larger than what most people would eat in a similar period of time under similar circumstances.

2. A sense of lack of control over eating during the episode (e.g., a feeling that one cannot stop eating or control what or how much one is eating).

B. The binge-eating episodes are associated with three (or more) of the following:

1. Eating much more rapidly than normal.

2. Eating until feeling uncomfortably full.

3. Eating large amounts of food when not feeling physically hungry.

4. Eating alone because of feeling embarrassed by how much one is eating.

5. Feeling disgusted with oneself, depressed, or very guilty afterward.

C. Marked distress regarding binge eating is present.

D. The binge eating occurs, on average, at least once a week for 3 months.

E. The binge eating is not associated with the recurrent use of inappropriate compensatory behavior as in bulimia nervosa and does not occur exclusively during the course of bulimia nervosa or anorexia nervosa.

Treatment

Counselling and certain medication, such as lisdexamfetamine and selective serotonin reuptake inhibitor (SSRIs), may help. Some recommend a multidisciplinary approach in the treatment of the disorder.

Counselling

Cognitive behavioral therapy (CBT) treatment has been demonstrated as a more effective form of treatment for BED than behavioral weight loss programs. 50 percent of BED individuals achieve complete remission from binge eating. CBT has also been shown to be an effective method to address self-image issues and psychiatric comorbidities (e.g., depression) associated with the disorder. Recent reviews have concluded that psychological interventions such as psychotherapy and behavioral interventions are more effective than pharmacological interventions for the treatment of binge eating disorder. There is the 12-step Overeaters Anonymous or Food Addicts in Recovery Anonymous.

Medication

Three other classes of medications are also used in the treatment of binge eating disorder: antidepressants, anticonvulsants, and anti-obesity medications. Antidepressant medications of the selective serotonin reuptake inhibitor (SSRI) class such as fluoxetine, fluvoxamine, or sertraline have been found to effectively reduce episodes of binge eating and reduce weight. Similarly, anticonvulsant medications such as topiramate and zonisamide may be able to effectively suppress appetite. The long-term effectiveness of medication for binge eating disorder is currently unknown.

Trials of antidepressants, anticonvulsants, and anti-obesity medications suggest that these medications are superior to placebo in reducing binge eating. Medications are not considered the treatment of choice because psychotherapeutic approaches, such as CBT, are more effective than medications for binge eating disorder. Medications also do not increase the effectiveness of psychotherapy, though some patients may benefit from anticonvulsant and anti-obesity medications, such as Phentermine/topiramate, for weight loss.

As of January 2015, lisdexamfetamine was the only drug approved by the Food and Drug Administration in the United States specifically for the treatment of binge eating.

Surgery

Bariatric surgery has also been proposed as another approach to treat BED and a recent meta-analysis showed that approximately two-thirds of individuals who seek this type of surgery for weight loss purposes have BED. Bariatric surgery recipients who had BED prior to receiving the surgery tend to have poorer weight-loss outcomes and are more likely to continue to exhibit eating behaviors characteristic of BED.

Prognosis

Individuals suffering from BED often have a lower overall quality of life and commonly experience social difficulties. Early behavior change is an accurate prediction of remission of symptoms later.

Individuals who have BED commonly have other comorbidities such as major depressive disorder, personality disorder, bipolar disorder, substance abuse, body dysmorphic disorder, kleptomania, irritable bowel syndrome, fibromyalgia, or an anxiety disorder. There may also be panic attacks and a history of attempted suicide.

While people of a healthy weight may overeat occasionally, an ongoing habit of consuming large amounts of food in a short period of time may ultimately lead to weight gain and obesity. Binging episodes usually include foods that are high in fat, sugar, and/or salt, but low in vitamins and minerals, as these types of foods tend to trigger greatest emotional reward. The main physical health consequences of this type of eating disorder are brought on by the weight gain resulting from the binging episodes. Up to 70% of individuals with BED may also be obese, and therefore obesity-associated morbidities such as high blood pressure and coronary artery disease type 2 diabetes mellitus gastrointestinal issues (e.g., gallbladder disease), high cholesterol levels, musculoskeletal problems and obstructive sleep apnea may also be present.

Epidemiology

The prevalence of BED in the general population is approximately 1-3%.

Binge eating disorder is the most common eating disorder in adults.

The limited amount of research that has been done on BED shows that rates of binge eating disorder are fairly comparable among men and women. The lifetime prevalence of binge eating disorder has been observed in studies to be 2.0 percent for men and 3.5 percent for women, higher than that of the commonly recognized eating disorders anorexia nervosa and bulimia nervosa.

Rates of binge eating disorder have also been found to be similar among black women, white women, and white men, while some studies have shown that binge eating disorder is more common among black women than among white women.

Though the research on binge eating disorders tends to be concentrated in North America, the disorder occurs across cultures, In the USA, BED is present in 0.8% of male adults and 1.6% of female adults in a given year.

Additionally, 30 to 40 percent of individuals seeking treatment for weight-loss can be diagnosed with binge eating disorder.

History, Society and Culture

The disorder was first described in 1959 by psychiatrist and researcher Albert Stunkard as "night eating syndrome" (NES). The term "binge eating" was coined to describe the same binging-type eating behavior but without the exclusive nocturnal component.

There is generally less research on binge eating disorder in comparison to anorexia nervosa and bulimia nervosa.

Orthorexia Nervosa

Orthorexia nervosa (also known as orthorexia) is a proposed eating disorder characterized by an excessive preoccupation with eating healthy food. The term was introduced in 1997 by American physician Steven Bratman, M.D. He suggested that some people's dietary restrictions intended to promote health may paradoxically lead to unhealthy consequences, such as social isolation, anxiety, loss of ability to eat in a natural, intuitive manner, reduced interest in the full range of other healthy human activities, and, in rare cases, severe malnutrition or even death.

In 2009, Ursula Philpot, chair of the British Dietetic Association and senior lecturer at Leeds Metropolitan University, described people with orthorexia nervosa as being "solely concerned with the quality of the food they put in their bodies, refining and restricting their diets according to their personal understanding of which foods are truly 'pure'." This differs from other eating disorders, such as anorexia nervosa and bulimia nervosa, where those affected focus on the quantity of food eaten.

"Orthorexia nervosa" is not recognized as an eating disorder by the American Psychiatric Association, and so is not mentioned as an official diagnosis in the widely used *Diagnostic and Statistical Manual of Mental Disorders* (DSM).

History

In a 1997 article in the magazine *Yoga Journal*, the American physician Steven Bratman coined the term "orthorexia nervosa" from the Greek (*ortho*, "right" or "correct"), and (*orexis*, "appetite"), literally meaning 'correct appetite', but in practice meaning 'correct diet'. The term is modeled on *anorexia*, literally meaning "without appetite", as used in the definition of the condition anorexia nervosa. (In both terms, "nervosa" indicates an unhealthy psychological state.) Bratman described orthorexia as an unhealthy fixation with what the individual considers to be healthy eating. Beliefs about what constitutes healthy eating commonly originate in one or another dietary theory such as raw foods veganism or macrobiotics, but are then taken to extremes, leading to disordered eating patterns and psychological and/or physical impairment. Bratman based this proposed condition on his personal experiences in the 1970s, as well as behaviors he observed among his patients in the 1990s. In 2000, Bratman, with David Knight, authored the book *Health Food Junkies*, which further expanded on the subject.

In 2015, responding to news articles in which the term orthorexia is applied to people who merely follow a non-mainstream theory of healthy eating, Bratman specified the following: "A theory may be conventional or unconventional, extreme or lax, sensible or totally wacky, but, regardless of the details, followers of the theory do not necessarily have orthorexia. They are simply adherents of a dietary theory. The term 'orthorexia' only applies when an eating disorder develops around that theory." Bratman elsewhere clarifies that with a few exceptions, most common theories of healthy eating are followed safely by the majority of their adherents; however, "for some people, going down the path of a restrictive diet in search of health may escalate into dietary perfectionism." Karin Kratina, PhD, writing for the National Eating Disorders Association, summarizes this process as follows: "Eventually food choices become so restrictive, in both variety and calories, that health suffers – an ironic twist for a person so completely dedicated to healthy eating."

Although orthorexia is not recognized as a mental disorder by the American Psychiatric Association, and it is not listed in the DSM-5, as of January 2016, four case reports and more than 40 other articles on the subject have been published in a variety of peer-reviewed journals internationally. According to a study published in 2011, two-thirds of a sample of 111 Dutch-speaking eating disorder specialists felt they had observed the syndrome in their clinical practice.

According to the *Macmillan English Dictionary,* the word is entering the English lexicon.

Diagnostic Criteria

In 2016, formal criteria for orthorexia were proposed in the peer-reviewed journal *Eating Behaviors* by authors Dr Thom Dunn of the University of Northern Colorado, and Steven Bratman. These criteria are as follows:

Criterion A. Obsessive focus on "healthy" eating, as defined by a dietary theory or set of beliefs whose specific details may vary; marked by exaggerated emotional distress in relationship to food choices perceived as unhealthy; weight loss may ensue, but this is conceptualized as an aspect of ideal health rather than as the primary goal. As evidenced by the following:

1. Compulsive behavior and/or mental preoccupation regarding affirmative and restrictive dietary practices believed by the individual to promote optimum health. (Footnotes to this criteria add: Dietary practices may include use of concentrated "food supplements." Exercise performance and/or fit body image may be regarded as an aspect or indicator of health.)

2. Violation of self-imposed dietary rules causes exaggerated fear of disease, sense of personal impurity and/or negative physical sensations, accompanied by anxiety and shame.

3. Dietary restrictions escalate over time, and may come to include elimination of entire food groups and involve progressively more frequent and/or severe "cleanses" (partial fasts) regarded as purifying or detoxifying. This escalation commonly leads to weight loss, but the desire to lose weight is absent, hidden or subordinated to ideation about healthy food.

Criterion B. The compulsive behavior and mental preoccupation becomes clinically impairing by any of the following:

1. Malnutrition, severe weight loss or other medical complications from restricted diet

2. Intrapersonal distress or impairment of social, academic or vocational functioning secondary to beliefs or behaviors about healthy diet

3. Positive body image, self-worth, identity and/or satisfaction excessively dependent on compliance with self-defined "healthy" eating behavior.

A diagnostic questionnaire has been developed for orthorexia sufferers, similar to questionnaires for other eating disorders, named the ORTO-15. However, the above cited article by Dunn and Bratman critiques this survey tool as lacking appropriate internal and external validation.

Symptoms

Symptoms of orthorexia nervosa include "obsessive focus on food choice, planning, purchase, preparation, and consumption; food regarded primarily as source of health rather than pleasure; distress or disgust when in proximity to prohibited foods; exaggerated faith that inclusion or elimination of particular kinds of food can prevent or cure disease or affect daily well-being; periodic shifts in dietary beliefs while other processes persist unchanged; moral judgment of others based on dietary choices; body image distortion around sense of physical "impurity" rather than weight; persistent belief that dietary practices are health-promoting despite evidence of malnutrition.".

Epidemiology

Results across scientific findings have yet to find a definitive conclusion to support whether nutrition students and professionals are at higher risk than other population subgroups, due to differing results in the research literature. There are only a few notable scientific works that, in an attempt to explore the breadth and depth of the still vaguely-understood illness, have tried to identify which groups in society are most vulnerable to its onset. This includes a 2008 German study, which based its research on the widespread suspicion that the most nutritionally-informed, such as university nutrition students, are a potential high-risk group for eating disorders, due to a substantial accumulation of knowledge on food and its relationship to health; the idea being that the more one knows about health, the more likely an unhealthy fixation about being healthy can develop. This study also inferred that orthorexic tendencies may even fuel a desire to study the science, indicating that many within this field might suffer from the disorder before commencing the course. However the results found that the students in the study, upon initial embarkation of their degree, did not have higher orthorexic values than other non-nutrition university students, and thus the report concluded that further research is needed to clarify the relationship between food-education and the onset of ON.

Similarly, in a Portuguese study on nutrition tertiary students, the participants' orthorexic scores (according to the ORTO-15 diagnostic questionnaire) actually decreased as they progressed through their course, as well as the overall risk of developing an eating disorder being an insignificant 4.2 percent. The participants also answered questionnaires to provide insight into their eating behaviours and attitudes, and despite this study finding that nutrition and health-science students tend to have more restrictive eating behaviours, these studies however found no evidence to support that these students have "more disturbed or disordered eating patterns than other students" These two aforementioned studies conclude that the more understanding of food one has is not necessarily a risk factor for ON, explaining that the data gathered suggests dietetics professionals are not at significant risk of it.

However, these epidemiologic studies have been critiqued as using a fundamentally flawed survey tool that inflates prevalence rates.

Media Reaction

The concept of orthorexia as a newly developing eating disorder has attracted significant media attention in the 21st century.

Biology

There has been no investigation into whether there may be a biological cause specific to orthorexia nervosa. It may be a food-centered manifestation of obsessive-compulsive disorder, which has a lot to do with control. A 2013 study of college students found that orthorexia severity was negatively associated with self-reported executive functioning. This means that the better the student did with cognitively complex tasks, including planning and decision-making, the less likely the student was to have orthorexia.

Muscle Dysmorphia

Muscle dysmorphia is the obsessive preoccupation with a delusional or exaggerated belief that one's own body is too small, too skinny, insufficiently muscular, or insufficiently lean, although in most cases, the individual's build is normal or even exceptionally large and muscular already. Sometimes called "bigorexia", "megarexia", or "reverse anorexia", it is a subtype of body dysmorphic disorder, but is often also grouped with eating disorders. Muscle dysmorphia mostly affects males, particularly those participating in athletics. They experience a disordered fixation on gaining body mass and often devote inordinate time and attention on exercise routines, dietary regimens, and nutritional supplements. The use of anabolic steroids is also common. Other body-dysmorphic preoccupations that are not muscle-dysmorphic are also usually present.

Muscle dysmorphia can be distressing, distracting, and debilitating disorder and can provoke absences from school, work, and socializing. When compared to other body dysmorphic disorders, rates of suicide attempts are especially high among people who have muscle dysmorphia. Although likened to anorexia nervosa in females, muscle dysmorphia is difficult to recognize, especially since males experiencing it typically look healthy to others.

The incidence of Muscle dysmorphia is rising, in part due to recent popularization of extreme cultural ideals of men's bodies.

History

Muscle dysmorphia was first conceptualized as a health risk in the late 1990s. Initially, the symptom profile was considered to be a reverse form of anorexia nervosa. Instead of a person desiring to be small and thin, he or she desires to be large and muscular. Later research, however, indicated that the subjective experience of muscle dysmorphia was more closely related to that of body dysmorphic disorder. This is still subject to debate.

Research has increased in recent years. As of 2016, 50% of all peer-reviewed studies on the topic had been published in the past 5 years. The American Psychiatric Association first recognized muscle dysmorphia as a valid disorder in 2013 in the fifth edition of the Diagnostic and Statistical Manual of Mental Disorders. In the DSM-5, it is classified as a specifier for body dysmorphic disorder. Muscle dysmorphia still remains absent from the International Statistical Classification of Diseases and Related Health Problems, the tenth issue of which was published in 1992.

Alternative Classifications

The classification of muscle dysmorphia has been widely debated and alternative DSM classifications have been proposed:

- Eating Disorder: Eating disorders and muscle dysmorphia share many characteristics. Many researchers have called for it to be reclassified as a type of eating disorder due to the fact that preoccupation with body weight and shape, and its modification, underpin both disorders. In general, body dysmorphic disorder does not typically include the food and exercise related psychopathology that characterize muscle dysmorphia and eating disorders. Studies have shown that people with muscle dysmorphia score higher on measures of eating disorders, such as the Eating Attitudes Test and Eating Disorder Inventory, than the general population. Also, individuals suffering from muscle dysmorphia and eating disorders typically experience high impairment while those suffering from body dysmorphia typically experience lower levels of impairment. There is even some evidence that treatment for eating disorders is effective for muscle dysmorphia as well. Muscle dysmorphia and anorexia nervosa share additional similarities such as diagnostic crossover with time and familial transmission. From a practical standpoint, it is possible that reclassifying muscle dysmorphia as an eating disorder would further reduce the size of the DSM's "Feeding and Eating Conditions Not Elsewhere Classified" section.

- Behavioral Addiction: Others have argued for muscle dysmorphia it to be reclassified as a behavioral addiction. It is argued that the addictive activity of muscle dysmorphia is the maintaining of body image through a number of different activities such as bodybuilding, exercise, eating and shopping for certain foods and food supplements, taking specific drugs, and purchasing and using physical exercise accessories. Although their activities may cause them harm, and may continue to cause them harm in the future, individuals with muscle dysmorphia continue to engage in them. This is similar to how people suffering from behavioral addictions still continue to engage in the harmful activities to which they are addicted. The typical behaviors that accompany muscle dysmorphia share many characteristics with behavioral addictions. For example, muscle building and dietary restriction in people who experience muscle dysmorphia hold high importance, can lead to mood modification, and can lead to interpersonal conflicts. People can build up tolerance to their muscle building and dietary restriction practices and may need to increase levels in order to achieve the desired physiological and/ or psychological effects. They can also experience symptoms of withdrawal if they are unable to engage in the maintenance activities and even if they are able to stop these activities, they are susceptible to relapse.

Signs and Symptoms

According to the DSM-5, muscle dysmorphia can be diagnosed if an individual meeting the diagnostic criteria for body dysmorphic disorder is "preoccupied with the idea that his or her body build is too small or insufficiently muscular." This specifier is still used even if the individual is preoccupied with other body areas, which is often the case.

Psychologists have expanded upon this basic framework and have found other clinical features often found in those with muscle dysmorphia. Individuals suffering from muscle dysmorphia are often consumed by activities aimed at increasing muscularity. This can often lead to participation in unhealthy behaviors (e.g. the use of physique-enhancing drugs, dietary restriction, and excessive exercise). People who suffer from muscle dysmorphia generally spend more than three hours per day thinking about becoming more muscular and believe that they have little control over their weightlifting activities. They engage in body monitoring and camouflaging behaviors, such as wearing multiple layers of clothing to appear larger.

These symptoms can be impairing. They experience severe distress regarding having their bodies viewed by others. They experience impaired occupational and social functioning and often report that their diet regimes interfere at least moderately with their lives. They often avoid activities, people, and places because of their embarrassment over their perceived lack of muscularity. Approximately 50% of patients have little or no insight into their condition and its severity.

They are also more likely to experience or have experienced a concurrent or past psychiatric diagnosis with eating disorders, mood disorders, anxiety disorders, and substance use disorder being the most common. They are more likely to have attempted suicide than members of the general population. Onset of muscle dysmorphia has been predicted to generally occur between 18 and 20 years of age.

Prevalence

Prevalence estimates for muscle dysmorphia have been highly variable, with estimates ranging anywhere from 1-54% of men being affected. Prevalence estimates are often found within more specific populations, with gym members, weightlifters, and bodybuilders showing higher prevalence rates than the general population. Even higher rates have been found among members of these groups who also use anabolic steroids. Onset of muscle dysmorphia has been predicted to generally occur between 18 and 20 years of age, but there may be significant prevalence rates in much younger populations since body dissatisfaction has been found in males as young as six years old. Muscle dysmorphia is far less common in women, but still possible, especially in women who are victims of sexual assault.

Cases cross cultural barriers, with clinical populations appearing in places such as China, South Africa, and Latin America. Prevalence in these countries may be mediated by exposure to western ideals of muscularity. One study found that college-aged men in Austria, France, and the United States report a similar gap between current perceived and ideal levels of muscularity. Meanwhile, populations that are less exposed to western ideals of muscularity tend to have lower prevalence rates.

Causes

The causes of muscle dysmorphia are unclear, but several significant risk factors and theories have been proposed:

- Muscle dysmorphia as a coping or defense mechanism: Many researchers have identified psychological predisposing factors associated with muscle dysmorphia. People suffering from muscle dysmorphia are more likely to have experienced or observed a traumatic event (e.g. sexual assault or domestic violence) than members of the general population. The drive to become muscular has been theorized to be a way for people to cope psychologically with past trauma. People suffering from muscle dysmorphia are also more likely to have been victimized, bullied, or ridiculed for perceived deficiencies (e.g. being small, weak, non-athletic, or intellectually inferior) as adolescents than the general population. It is theorized that many of these people are driven to become more muscular because it would not only help them cope with their unpleasant past, but it would also allow them to defend themselves in the future or at least stop the harassment.

- Muscle dysmorphia as a result of low self-esteem and insecurities: Low self-esteem can contribute to muscle dysmorphia, with lower levels being linked to higher body dissatisfaction and higher levels of muscle dysmorphia Individuals who develop beliefs that muscular appearance is important and have lower perceptions of themselves are at a heightened risk for developing muscle dysmorphia. For people whose self-esteem is contingent upon appearance, this association is even more dangerous as they tend to spend even more time on appearance-related behaviors, such as lifting weights. Muscle preoccupations may also develop as a way to address insecurities, such as insecurity about sexual capability. Research has found a link between muscularity and feelings of reproductive success and have postulated that for people suffering from Muscle Dysmorphia, muscles may become a secondary sex characteristic, which indicate virility and the ability to provide safety and resources for partners and offspring. Drive for muscularity is also correlated negatively with genital satisfaction, indicating that some men may develop muscularity preoccupations as a way to compensate for perceived deficiencies.

- The negative effects of media exposure and muscle dysmorphia: Other research has pointed towards the threat of popular culture and media exposure. Not only does media in western culture promote standards of attractiveness, but marketing campaigns have also begun to specifically target male body-image insecurities. This generates social comparison and pressure for individuals to take measures to conform to the ideal. Men exposed to muscular images show a significantly greater discrepancy between their own level muscularity and desired level of muscularity than men who are not exposed to muscular images. Unfortunately, the number of fitness magazines directed at men and the number of partially-clothed well-muscled men in magazine advertisements have increased over the past 20 years, increasing the potential for men to be exposed to these images. Studies have found that the strongest predictor of a drive for muscularity in college aged men is the extent to which they have internalized the ideal male body presented by the media.

- Participation in sports and Muscle Dysmorphia: A correlation has also been found between sports participation and muscle dysmorphia. The condition has been found to be positively correlated with involvement in sports such as football and wrestling – sports that emphasize size and strength and in which being large carries the notion of gaining an "edge" over the competition. Sports can help expose individuals to the social ideal of muscularity and reinforce the obtainment and maintenance of this ideal. In general, athletes are more critical of their bodies and body weight than those who do not regularly engage in planned exercise. Athletes who are both critical of their bodies and fail to achieve performance standards may resort to the extreme measures associated with muscle dysmorphia to achieve a body ideal. Athletes share many of the psychological factors that have been theorized to increase the likelihood of muscle dysmorphia such as high levels of competitiveness, high need for control, and perfectionist tendencies. It is unclear if the sports serve as a gateway to muscle dysmorphia or if those predisposed to the condition are more likely to participate in such sports.

Treatment

Treatment of muscle dysmorphia is complicated by the fact that many individuals who suffer from it do not recognize it or seek treatment. It becomes the responsibility of healthcare professionals to identify the problem and intervene at the correct time. The first step is convincing the individual that he or she needs help. Unfortunately, scientific research on the treatment of muscle dysmorphia is severely limited and largely based on anecdotes and case reports. No specific treatment programs have been developed although several general approaches have been successful. Some research has supported the efficacy of family-based therapy, cognitive behavioural therapy, and the use of selective serotonin reuptake inhibitor (anti-depressant) medications in the treatment of muscle dysmorphia. Like research on treatment, research on prognosis has been severely limited

Diabulimia

Diabulimia (a portmanteau of *diabetes* and *bulimia*) refers to an eating disorder in which people with Type 1 diabetes deliberately give themselves less insulin than they need, for the purpose of weight loss. Diabulimia is not currently recognized as a formal diagnosis by the medical or psychiatric communities. However, the phrases "disturbed eating behavior" or "disordered eating behavior" (DEB in both cases), or disordered eating (DE) are quite common in medical and psychiatric literature which addresses the condition of patients who have Type 1 diabetes and who also intentionally manipulate insulin doses to control weight along with bulimic behavior.

Symptoms

A person with diabulimia, especially if not treated early, can suffer negative effects on the body earlier than one who is managing properly. Of diabetics who have a DEB, some intentionally misuse insulin as a means to control weight.

Suspension of insulin, combined with overeating and resulting in ketoacidosis. Multiple hospitalizations for ketoacidosis or hyperglycemia are cues to screen for an underlying emotional conflict.

Short term

These are the short term symptoms of patients with diabulimia

- Constant urination
- Constant thirst
- Excessive appetite
- High blood glucose levels (often over 600 mg/dL or 33 mmol/L)
- Weakness
- Fatigue
- Large amounts of glucose in the urine
- Inability to concentrate
- Electrolyte disturbance
- Severe ketonuria, and, in DKA, severe ketonemia

- Low sodium levels

Medium term

These are the medium term symptoms of patients with diabulimia. They are prevalent when diabulimia has not been treated and hence also includes the short term symptoms

- Muscle atrophy

- GERD

- Indigestion

- Severe weight loss

- Proteinuria

- Moderate to severe dehydration

- Edema with fluid replacement

- High cholesterol

Long term

If a person with Type 1 diabetes who has diabulimia suffers from the disease for more than a short time—usually due to alternating phases during which insulin is injected properly, and relapses, during which they have diabulimia—then the following longer-term symptoms can be expected:

- Severe kidney damage - high blood sugar can overwork the kidneys, eventually leading to kidney failure and the need for a kidney transplant

- Severe neuropathy (nerve damage to hands and feet)

- Extreme fatigue

- Edema (during blood sugars controlled phases)

- Heart problems

- High cholesterol

- Osteoporosis

- Death

Often, people with Type 1 diabetes who omit insulin injections will have already been diagnosed with an eating disorder such as anorexia nervosa, bulimia nervosa These individuals are often not aware that diabulimia is more common than they think and is also very difficult to overcome. Unlike anorexia and bulimia, diabulimia sometimes requires the afflicted individual to stop caring for a medical condition. Unlike vomiting or starving, there is sometimes no clear action or willpower involved. Diabulimia may be more appealing to individuals who want to lose weight.

Many articles and studies further conclude that diabetic females have, on average, higher body mass index (BMI) than do their nondiabetic counterparts. Girls and young adult woman with higher BMIs are also shown to be more likely to have disordered eating behavior (DEB). Many authoritative articles have been published which show that preteen and teenage girls with Type 1 diabetes have significantly higher rates of eating disorders of all types than do girls without diabetes. This condition can be triggered or exacerbated by the need for diabetics to exercise constant vigilance in regard to food, weight and glycemic control. In adolescent females, increased weight gain that insulin treatment can cause may play roles in the increased risk for onset of anorexia and/or bulimia.

Treatment

There are no specific guidelines for the treatment of diabetes and disordered eating, but the standard approach for treatment of two complex conditions as multidisciplinary team of professionals which in this case could include an endocrinologist, psychiatrist, psychologist, dietician, etc.

Drunkorexia

Drunkorexia is a colloquialism for self-imposed starvation or binge eating/purging combined with alcohol abuse. The term is generally used to denote the utilisation of extreme weight control methods (such as the aforementioned starvation or purging) as a tool to compensate for planned binge drinking.

Research on the combination of an eating disorder and binge drinking has primarily focused on the patterns of college-aged women, but the phenomenon has also been noted among young men. Studies show that college students engage in this combination of self-imposed malnutrition and binge drinking to avoid weight gain from alcohol. A study by the University of Missouri found that 30% of female college students admitted that within the last year they had restricted food in order to consume greater quantities of alcohol. The same study found that men are more likely engage in similar behavior in order to save money for purchasing alcohol. According to the study, 67% of students who restrict calories prior to alcoholic beverage consumption do so to prevent weight gain, while 21% did so to facilitate alcohol intoxication.

According to the Eating Disorder Center of Denver, of the participating college-aged females in an adjunct research study, about 75% met the criteria for alcohol abuse.

'Showbuzz', a CBS news site, has broadcast that, "Drunkorexia is a media coined term reflecting an alarmingly real trend among young women. The non-medical slang term refers to women who choose to eat less so they can party without gaining weight."

R. Andrew Chambers, MD, Assistant Professor, Institute of Psychiatric Research and Director, Laboratory for Translational Neuroscience of Dual Diagnosis Disorders notes that many celebrity blog sites report similar patterns of behavior among young actresses such as Lindsay Lohan and Paris Hilton, and that the condition could be mimicked within the entertainment industry and contemporary youth culture at large.

History of Binge Drinking and Eating Disorders among College Students

A 2002 study from O'Malley and Johnston reviewed data from the national College Alcohol Study, the Core Institute, Monitoring the Future, and the National College Health Risk Behavior Survey affirming that 70% of participating college students reported consuming alcohol within the prior month and 40% had engaged in binge drinking. First-year college students have been identified as uniquely predisposed to binge drinking.

According to disclosure from the National Eating Disorder Association in 2006, approximately 20% of college students, both male and female, admitted to suffering from an eating disorder at some point in their life. Clinical eating disorders encompass binge eating, chronic dieting, fasting or purging and the use of laxatives to control weight. Furthermore, first-year college students are predisposed to eating disorders as an attempt to avoid the fabled "Freshman 15," weight gain that results from adjusting to a college lifestyle.

A study was conducted in 2010 at a Southeastern University, using 692 freshmen. This study examined caloric restriction among students prior to planned alcohol consumption. These results indicated that 99 of 695 (14%) of first year (freshmen) students reported restricting calories prior to drinking. 6% reported this behaviour to avoid weight gain.

A 2001 CASA report estimated that 30-50% of individuals with bulimia and 12-18% of individuals with anorexia had previously abused or were currently dependent on alcohol. 35% of those with alcohol or drug dependency reported a concurrent eating disorder. Results demonstrated a clear correlation between individual histories of eating disorders and binge drinking and/or alcohol dependence.

A survey was conducted in 2013, using 107 female University students, to study the frequency and correlates of self-induced vomiting after consuming alcohol. The results showed that 59.8% of the participants who reported drinking alcohol, also appeared to have engaged in self-induced vomiting after alcohol consumption. Participants that reported self-induced vomiting after alcohol consumption, also reported more bulimia nervosa symptomatology.

In an Australian context, a study was undertaken in 2013 that surveyed 139 Australian women, aged between 18 and 29, who were enrolled in an undergraduate degree at university. These women were asked to complete a survey regarding compensatory eating and behaviours in response to alcohol consumption to test for 'Drunkorexia' symptomatology. In the sample tested, 79% of participants demonstrated engaging in characterised Drunkorexia behaviour. Further analysis of the results showed that social norms of drinking and the social norms associated with body image and thinness impacted heavily upon the motivation for these behaviours.

Another study undertaken in 2012 showed that there exists a further correlation between college students who are very physically active and alcohol dependence. Excessive exercise is often perceived as a symptom of Anorexia Nervosa (and other associated eating disorders) which further exemplifies the existence of 'Drunkorexia', particularly in college age individuals. The study showed that those individuals who were more physically active than their peers had a higher tendency to be alcohol dependent or to engage in regular binge drinking.

The National Association of Anorexia Nervosa and Associated Disorders reports that 72% of women who admit to alcohol abuse also classify as suffering from an eating disorder.

Link between Binge Drinking and Eating Disorders

There appears to be a link between eating disorders and substance abuse, with studies revealing people experiencing an eating disorder are at a higher risk of developing substance abuse problems.

According to the National Institutes of Health, 1 in 6 people in the US have a drinking problem and approximately 10 million Americans are believed to suffer from potentially life-threatening eating disorders.

Furthermore, those who suffer from drunkorexia, have a greater likelihood of developing a more serious eating disorder. A previous report published in the American journal 'Biological Psychiatry' found that up to one third of bulimics struggle with alcohol or drug abuse.

A report in the U.S examining the relationship between eating disorders and substance abuse revealed that anorexia and bulimia are the eating disorders most commonly linked to substance abuse, and up to half of the people with eating disorders abuse alcohol or illicit drugs. Shared Risk Factors: -occur in times of transition or stress -common brain chemistry -common family history -low self-esteem, depression, anxiety, impulsivity History of sexual or physical abuse -unhealthy parental behaviours and low monitoring of children's activities -Unhealthy peer norms and social pressures -Susceptibility to messages from advertising and entertainment media

Symptoms of Drunkorexia

Drunkorexia consists of 3 major aspects: alcohol use/abuse, food intake restriction, and excessive physical activity. It is commonly summarised in the following activities:

- Counting daily calorie intake (commonly known as "calorie counting") to ensure no weight will be gained when consuming alcohol.

- Missing or skipping meals to conserve calories for consumption of alcoholic beverages.

- Over exercising to counterweigh for calories consumed from alcoholic beverages.

- Consuming an extreme amount of alcohol to vomit previously digested food.

Treatment of Drunkorexia

Drunkorexia is not a medically diagnosed disorder therefore there is no specific treatment. However, as drunkorexia is a combination of two different disorders, binge drinking and eating disorders such as anorexia and bulimia the treatment will need to address both.

Effects of Drunkorexia

The combination of self-starvation and alcohol abuse can lead to an array of physical and psychological consequences. For example, drinking in a state of malnutrition can predispose individuals to a higher rate of blackouts, alcohol poisoning, alcohol-related injury, violence, or illness. Drinking on an empty stomach allows ethanol to reach the blood system at a swifter pace and raises one's blood alcohol content with an often dangerous speed. This can render the drinker more vulnerable to alcohol-related brain damage. In addition, alcohol abuse can have a detrimental impact on hydration and the body's retention of minerals and nutrients, further exacerbating the consequences of malnutrition and denigrating an individual's cognitive faculties. This can ultimately have a negative impact on academic performance.

These harmful consequences can be more easily induced in women, as women are oftentimes less capable of metabolizing alcohol than men. On CBS News, Carrie Wilkins, PhD, of the Center for Motivation and Change (a private practice group based in New York City) describes how women are more vulnerable to particular toxic side effects of alcohol consumption.

Drunkorexia can lead to short term and long term cognitive problems including difficulty concentrating and difficulty making decisions. It also increases the risk of developing more serious eating disorders or alcohol abuse problems. As binge drinking is involved there is a greater risk for violence, risky sexual behavior, alcohol poisoning, substance abuse and chronic disease later in life.

Who is at Most Risk

Drunkorexia is found to be most common among university students who are faced with the conflicting pressure of heavy drinking and maintaining a slim physique. Researchers from the University of Missouri who questioned college students found that 16% of those surveyed reported restricting calories to save them for drinking. This practice of restricting calories for drinking was found to be three times more common in woman than men.

Motivations for Drunkorexia

The motivations behind Drunkorexia as a pattern of behaviour is one of the lesser understood aspects of the condition. It is suspected that the predominant factors in the development of Drunkorexia are a distorted self perception congruent with unrealistic standards of body image, peer pressure to assimilate to the norm in terms of social drinking and societal standards of beauty, as a coping mechanism for anxiety and depression and as a means of getting intoxicated rapidly in response to stress and or peer pressure.

A study undertaken in 1983 sought to investigate if individuals who regularly participated in binge drinking, or were alcohol dependent, had a more distorted self perception than those individuals who were not abusing alcohol. The study measured the relative rate of body image distortion by asking participants in both a control, non-alcoholic abusive group and a group of alcohol dependent individuals to estimate the length and width of 22 different body parts, including the shoulders, arms, chest etc. The results showed that those individuals who were alcohol abusers saw their body parts as much larger than they actually were, indicating a distorted perception of self. The results from this study indicate that there may be a link between those who are predispositioned to engage in alcohol dependant or binge drinking behavior and a distorted perception of self which would help psychiatrists and clinical practitioners establish an at risk population and further would aid in better understanding and treating Drunkorexia.

Other motivations for drunkorexia include; preventing weight gain, saving money that would be spent on food to buy alcohol, and getting intoxicated faster which also saves money as they won't need to buy as many drinks.

Drunkorexia as a Diagnosis

Co-existing, and self-reinforcing starvation and alcohol disorders are gaining recognition in the fields of dual diagnosis, psychiatry, and addictionology.

Other Specified Feeding or Eating Disorder

Other specified feeding or eating disorder or OSFED is the *DSM-5* category that replaces the category formerly called Eating Disorder Not Otherwise Specified (EDNOS) in *DSM-IV*, and that captures feeding disorders and eating disorders of clinical severity that do not meet diagnostic criteria for anorexia nervosa (AN), bulimia nervosa (BN), binge eating disorder (BED), avoidant/restrictive food intake disorder (ARFID), pica, or rumination disorder. OSFED includes five examples: atypical AN, BN (of low frequency and/or limited duration), BED (of low frequency and/or limited duration), purging disorder, and night eating syndrome (NES).

Characteristics

The five OSFED examples that can be considered eating disorders include atypical AN, BN (of low frequency and/or limited duration), BED (of low frequency and/or limited duration), purging disorder, and NES. Of note, OSFED is not limited to these five examples, and can include individuals with heterogeneous eating disorder presentations (i.e., OSFED-other). Another term, Unspecified Feeding or Eating Disorder (UFED), is used to describe individuals for whom full diagnostic criteria are not met but the reason remains unspecified or the clinician does not have adequate information to make a more definitive diagnosis.

- Atypical Anorexia Nervosa: In atypical AN, individuals meet all of the criteria for AN, with the exception of the weight criterion: the individual's weight remains within or above the normal range, despite significant weight loss.

- Atypical Bulimia Nervosa: In this sub-threshold version of BN, individuals meet all criteria for BN, with the exception of the frequency criterion: binge eating and inappropriate compensatory behaviors occur, on average, less than once a week and/or for fewer than 3 months.

- Binge-eating disorder (of low frequency and/or limited duration): In this sub-threshold version of BED, individuals must meet all criteria for BED, with the exception of the frequency criterion: binge eating occurs, on average, less than once a week and/or for fewer than 3 months.

- Purging Disorder: In purging disorder, purging behavior aimed to influence weight or shape is present, but in the absence of binge eating.

- Night Eating Syndrome: In NES, individuals have recurrent episodes of eating at night, such as eating after awakening from sleep or excess calorie intake after the evening meal. This eating behavior is not culturally acceptable by group norms, such as the occasional late-night munchies after a gathering. NES includes an awareness and recall of the eating, is not better explained by external influences such as changes in the individual's sleep-wake cycle, and causes significant distress and/or impairment of functioning. Though not defined specifically in *DSM-5*, research criteria for this diagnosis proposed adding the following criteria (1) the consumption of at least 25% of daily caloric intake after the evening meal and/or (2) evening awakenings with ingestions at least twice per week.

Epidemiology

Few studies to date have examined OSFED prevalence. The largest community study is by Stice (2013), who examined 496 adolescent females who completed annual diagnostic interviews over 8 years. Lifetime prevalence by age 20 for OSFED overall was 11.5%. 2.8% had atypical AN, 4.4% had subthreshold BN, 3.6% had subthreshold BED, and 3.4% had purging disorder. Peak age of onset for OSFED was 18–20 years. NES was not assessed in this study, but estimates from other studies suggest that it presents in 1% of the general population.

A few studies have compared the prevalence of EDNOS and OSFED and found that though the prevalence of atypical eating disorders decreased with the new classification system, the prevalence still remains high. For example, in a population of 215 young patients presenting for ED treatment, the diagnosis of EDNOS to OSFED decreased from 62.3% to 32.6%. In another study of 240 females in the U.S. with a lifetime history of an eating disorder, the prevalence changed from 67.9% EDNOS to 53.3% OSFED. Although the prevalence appears to reduce when using the categorizations of EDNOS vs. OSFED, a high proportion of cases still receive diagnoses of atypical eating disorders, which creates difficulties in communication, treatment planning, and basic research.

Treatment

Few studies guide the treatment of individuals with OSFED. However, cognitive behavioral therapy (CBT), which focuses on the interplay between thoughts, feelings, and behaviors, has been shown to be the leading evidence-based treatment for the eating disorders of BN and BED. For OSFED, a particular cognitive behavioral treatment can be used called CBT-Enhanced (CBT-E), which was designed to treat all forms of eating disorders. This method focuses not only what is thought to be the central cognitive disturbance in eating disorders (i.e., over-evaluation of eating, shape, and weight), but also on modifying the mechanisms that sustain eating disorder psychopathology, such as perfectionism, core low self-esteem, mood intolerance, and interpersonal difficulties. CBT-E showed effectiveness in two studies (total N = 219) and well maintained over 60-week follow-up periods. CBT-E is not specific to individual types of eating disorders but is based on the concept that common mechanisms are involved in the persistence of atypical eating disorders, AN, and BN.

History

In 1980, *DSM-III* was the first *DSM* to include a category for eating disorders that could not be classified in the categories of AN, BN, or pica. This category was called Atypical Eating Disorder. Atypical Eating Disorder was described in one sentence in the *DSM-III* and received very little attention in the literature, as it was perceived to be uncommon compared to the other defined eating disorders. In *DSM-III-R*, published in 1987, the Atypical Eating Disorder category became known as Eating Disorder Not Otherwise Specified (EDNOS). *DSM-III-R* included examples of individuals who would meet criteria for EDNOS, in part to acknowledge the increasingly recognized heterogeneity of individuals within the diagnostic category.

In 1994, *DSM-IV* was published and expanded EDNOS to include six clinical presentations. These presentations included individuals who:

- met criteria for AN, but continued to menstruate,

- met criteria for AN, but still had weight in the normal range despite significant weight loss,

- met criteria for BN but did not meet frequency criterion for binge eating or purging,

- engaged in inappropriate compensatory behavior after eating small amounts of food, or

- repeatedly chewed or spit out food, or who binged on food but did not subsequently purge.

A disadvantage of *DSM-IV*'s broad EDNOS category was that people with very different symptoms were still classified as having the same diagnosis, making it difficult to access care specific to the disorder and conduct research on the diversity of pathology within EDNOS. Furthermore, EDNOS was perceived as less severe than AN or BN, despite findings that individuals diagnosed with ED-NOS share similarities with full-threshold AN or BN in the degree of eating pathology, general psychopathology, and physical health. This perception prevented people in need from seeking help or insurance companies from covering treatment costs. *DSM-5*, published in 2013, sought to address these issues by adding new diagnoses and revising existing criteria

Feeding Disorder

A feeding disorder in infancy or early childhood is a child's refusal to eat certain food groups, textures, solids or liquids for a period of at least one month, which causes the child to not gain enough weight, grow naturally, or cause any developmental delays. Feeding disorders resemble failure to thrive, except that at times in feeding disorder there is no medical or physiological condition that can explain the very small amount of food the children consume or their lack of growth. Some of the times a previous medical condition that has been resolved is causing the issue.

Symptoms

Children attempting to swallow different food textures often vomit, gag, or choke while eating. At feeding times they may react negatively to attempts to feed them, and refuse to eat. Other symptoms include head turns, crying, difficulty in chewing or vomiting and spitting whilst eating. Many children may have feeding difficulties and may be picky eaters, but most of them still have a fairly healthy diet. Children with a feeding disorder however, will completely abandon some of the food groups, textures, or liquids that are necessary for human growth and development

Children with this disorder can develop much more slowly because of their lack of nutritional intake. In severe cases the child seems to feel socially isolated because of the lack of social activities involving foods.

Types

Feeding disorder has been divided into six further sub-types:

1. Feeding disorder of state regulation

2. Feeding disorder of reciprocity (neglect)

3. Infantile anorexia

4. Sensory food aversion

5. Feeding disorder associated with concurrent medical condition

6. Post-traumatic feeding disorder

Associated Problems

A few of the medical and psychological conditions that have been known to be associated with this disorder include:

• Gastrointestinal motility disorders

• Oral-motor dysfunction

• Failure to thrive

• Prematurity

• Food allergies

• Sensory problems

• Reflux

• Feeding tube placement

A child that is suffering from malnutrition can have permanently stunted mental and physical development. Getting treatment early is essential and can prevent many of the complications. They can also develop further eating disorders later in life such as anorexia nervosa, or they could become a limited eater—though they could still be a healthy child they may become a picky eater.

Diagnosis

A barium swallow test is often performed, where the child is given a liquid or food with barium in it. This allows the consulting medical practitioners to trace the swallow-function on an X-ray or other investigative system such as a CAT scan. An endoscopic assignment test can also be performed, where an endoscope is used to view the oesophagus and throat on a screen. It can also allow viewing of how the patient will react during feeding.

Treatments

There is no quick cure, and treatment will be based on what problems may be causing the feeding disorder. Depending on the condition, the following steps can be taken: increasing the number of foods that are accepted, increasing the amount of calories and the amount of fluids; checks for vitamin or mineral deficiencies; finding out what the illnesses or psychosocial problems are. To accomplish these goals patients may have to be hospitalized for extensive periods of time. Treatment involves professionals from multiple fields of study including, but not limited to; behavior analysts (Behavioral interventions), occupational and speech therapist who specialize in feeding disorders, dietitians, psychologists and physician. To obtain the best results, treatment should include a behavior modification plan under the guidance of multiple professionals. If the child has oral motor difficulties related to the feeding disorder a pediatric occupational or speech therapist who is trained in feeding disorders and oral motor function should help develop a plan.

Epidemiology

Some 25% to 40% of infants and children are reported to have feeding problems—mainly colic, vomiting, slow feeding, and refusal to eat. It has been reported that up to 80% of infants with developmental handicaps also demonstrate feeding problems while 1 to 2% of infants aged less than one year show severe food refusal and poor growth. Among infants born prematurely, 40% to 70% experience some form of feeding problem.

Avoidant/Restrictive Food Intake Disorder

Avoidant/restrictive food intake disorder (ARFID), also previously known as selective eating disorder (SED), is a type of eating disorder, as well as feeding disorder, where the consumption of certain foods is limited based on the food's appearance, smell, taste, texture, brand, presentation, or a past negative experience with the food.

Definition

The fifth edition of the *Diagnostic and Statistical Manual of Mental Disorders* (DSM-5) renamed "Feeding Disorder of Infancy or Early Childhood" to Avoidant/Restrictive Food Intake Disorder, and broadened the diagnostic criteria. Previously defined as a disorder exclusive to children and adolescents, the DSM-5 broadened the disorder to include adults who limit their eating and are affected by related physiological or psychological problems, but who do not fall under the definition of another eating disorder.

The DSM-5 defines the following diagnostic criteria:

- Disturbance in eating or feeding, as evidenced by one or more of:

    o   Substantial weight loss (or, in children, absence of expected weight gain)

    o   Nutritional deficiency

    o   Dependence on a feeding tube or dietary supplements

    o   Significant psychosocial interference

- Disturbance not due to unavailability of food, or to observation of cultural norms

- Disturbance not due to anorexia nervosa or bulimia nervosa, and no evidence of disturbance in experience of body shape or weight

- Disturbance not better explained by another medical condition or mental disorder, or when occurring concurrently with another condition, the disturbance exceeds what is normally caused by that condition

In previous years, the DSM was not inclusive in recognizing all of the challenges associated with feeding and eating disorders in 3 main domains:

- Eating Disorders Not Otherwise Specified (EDNOS) was an all-inclusive, placeholder group for all individuals that presented challenges with feeding

- The category of Feeding Disorder of Infancy/ Early Childhood was noted to be too broad, limiting specification when treating these behaviors

- There are children and youth who present feeding challenges but do not fit within any existing categories to date

Children are often picky eaters, this does not necessarily mean they meet the criteria for an ARFID diagnosis. In addition, self-identification as having ARFID may contribute to ARFID.

Signs and Symptoms

Sufferers of ARFID have an inability to eat certain foods. "Safe" foods may be limited to certain food types and even specific brands. In some cases, afflicted individuals will exclude whole food groups, such as fruits or vegetables. Sometimes excluded foods can be refused based on color. Some may only like very hot or very cold foods, very crunchy or hard-to-chew foods, or very soft foods, or avoid sauces.

Most sufferers of ARFID will still maintain a healthy or normal body weight. There are no specific outward appearances associated with ARFID. Sufferers can experience physical gastrointestinal reactions to adverse foods such as retching, vomiting or gagging. Some studies have identified symptoms of social avoidance due to their eating habits. Most, however, would change their eating habits if they could.

Comorbidity

The determination of the cause of ARFID has been difficult due to the lack of diagnostic criteria and concrete definition. However, many have proposed other mental disorders that are comorbid with ARFID.

There are different kinds of 'sub-categories' identified for ARFID:

- Sensory-based avoidance, where the individual refuse food intake based on smell, texture, color, brand, presentation

- A lack of interest in consuming the food, or tolerating it nearby

- Food being associated with fear-evoking stimuli that have developed through a learned history

ARFID and Autism

Symptoms of ARFID are usually found with symptoms of other disorders. Some form of feeding disorder is found in 80% of children that also have a developmental disability. Children often exhibit symptoms of obsessive-compulsive disorder and autism. Although many people with ARFID have symptoms of these disorders, they usually do not qualify for a full diagnosis. Strict behavior patterns and difficulty adjusting to new things are common symptoms in patients that are on the autistic spectrum. A study done by Schreck at Pennsylvania State University compared the eating habits of children with ASD and typically developing children. After analyzing their eating patterns, they suggested that the children with some degree of ASD have a higher degree of selective eating. These children were found to have similar patterns of selective eating and favored more energy dense foods such as nuts and whole grains. Eating a diet of energy dense foods could put these children at a greater risk for health problems such as obesity and other chronic diseases due to the high fat and low fiber content of energy dense foods. Due to the tie to ASD, children are less likely to outgrow their selective eating behaviors and most likely should meet with a clinician to address their eating issues.

ARFID as an Anxiety Disorder

Specific food avoidances could be caused by food phobias that cause great anxiety when a person is presented with new or feared foods. Most eating disorders are related to a fear of gaining weight. Those who suffer from ARFID do not have this fear, but the psychological symptoms and anxiety created is similar.

Clinical Diagnosis

Clinicians will often follow a diagnostic checklist to test whether or not an individual is exhibiting behaviors and characteristics that may lead to a diagnosis of ARFID. Clinicians will look at the variety of foods an individual consumes, as well as the portion size of accepted foods. They will also question how long the avoidance or refusal of particular foods has lasted, and if there are any associated medical concerns, such as malnutrition.

Treatment

For Adults

With time the symptoms of ARFID can lessen and can eventually disappear without treatment. However, in some cases treatment will be needed as the symptoms persist into adulthood. The most common type of treatment for ARFID is some form of cognitive-behavioral therapy. Working with a clinician can help to change behaviors more quickly than symptoms may typically disappear without treatment. Also hypnotherapy may be used. In that it lessens the anxiety associated with food.

There are support groups for adults with ARFID.

For Children

Children can benefit from a four stage in-home treatment program based on the principles of systematic desensitization. The four stages of the treatment are record, reward, relax and review.

- In the record stage, children are encouraged to keep a log of their typical eating behaviors without attempting to change their habits as well as their cognitive feelings.

- The reward stage involves systematic desensitization. Children create a list of foods that they might like to try eating some day. These foods may not be drastically different from their normal diet, but perhaps a familiar food prepared in a different way. Because the goal is for the children to try new foods, children are rewarded when they sample new foods.

- The relaxation stage is most important for those children that suffer severe anxiety when presented with unfavorable foods. Children learn to relax to reduce the anxiety that they feel. Children work through a list of anxiety-producing stimuli and can create a story line with relaxing imagery and scenarios. Often these stories can also include the introduction of new foods with the help of a real person or fantasy person. Children then listen to this story before eating new foods as a way to imagine themselves participating in an expanded variety of foods while relaxed.

- The final stage, review, is important to keep track of the child's progress. It is important to include both one-on-one sessions with the child, as well as with the parent in order to get a clear picture of how the child is progressing and if the relaxation techniques are working.

Night Eating Syndrome

Night eating syndrome (NES) is an eating disorder, characterized by a delayed circadian pattern of food intake. Although there is some degree of comorbidity with binge eating disorder, it differs from binge eating in that the amount of food consumed in the evening/night is not necessarily objectively large nor is a loss of control over food intake required. It was originally described by Dr. Albert Stunkard in 1955 and is currently included in the other specified feeding or eating disorder category of the DSM-5. Research diagnostic criteria have been proposed and include evening hyperphagia (consumption of 25% or more of the total daily calories after the evening meal) and/or nocturnal awakening and ingestion of food two or more times per week. The person must have awareness of the night eating to differentiate it from the parasomnia sleep-related eating disorder (SRED). Three of five associated symptoms must also be present: lack of appetite in the morning, urges to eat in the evening/at night, belief that one must eat in order to fall back to sleep at night, depressed mood, and/or difficulty sleeping.

NES affects both men and women, between 1 and 2% of the general population, and approximately 10% of obese individuals. The age of onset is typically in early adulthood (spanning from late teenage years to late twenties) and is often long-lasting, with children rarely reporting NES. People with NES have been shown to have higher scores for depression and low self-esteem, and it has been demonstrated that nocturnal levels of the hormones melatonin and leptin are decreased. The relationship between NES and the parasomnia SRED is in need of further clarification. There is debate as to whether these should be viewed as separate diseases, or part of a continuum. Consuming foods containing serotonin has been suggested to aid in the treatment of NES, but other research indicates that diet by itself cannot appreciably raise serotonin levels in the brain. A few foods (for example, bananas) contain serotonin, but they do not affect brain serotonin levels, and various foods contain tryptophan, but the extent to which they affect brain serotonin levels must be further explored scientifically before conclusions can be drawn, and "the idea, common in popular culture, that a high-protein food such as turkey will raise brain tryptophan and serotonin is, unfortunately, false."

Comorbidities

NES is sometimes comorbid with excess weight; as many as 28% of individuals seeking gastric bypass surgery were found to suffer from NES in one study. However, not all individuals with NES are overweight. Night eating has been associated with diabetic complications. Many people with NES also experience depressed mood and anxiety disorders.

Nocturnal Sleep-related Eating Disorder

Nocturnal sleep-related eating disorder (NSRED), also known as sleep-related eating disorder (SRED), sleep eating, or somnambulistic eating, is a combination of a parasomnia and an eating disorder. It is described as being in a specific category within somnambulism or a state of sleepwalking that includes behaviors connected to a person's conscious wishes or wants. Thus many times NSRED is a person's fulfilling of their conscious wants that they suppress; however, this disorder is difficult to distinguish from other similar types of disorders.

NSRED is closely related to Night Eating Syndrome (NES) except for the fact that those suffering from NES are completely awake and aware of their eating and bingeing at night while those suffering from NSRED are sleeping and unaware of what they are doing. NES is primarily considered an eating disorder while NSRED is primarily considered a parasomnia; however, both are a combination of parasomnia and eating disorders since those suffering from NES usually have insomnia or difficulty sleeping and those suffering from NSRED experience symptoms similar to binge eating. Some even argue over whether NES and NSRED are the same or distinct disorders. Even though there have been debates over these two disorders, specialists have examined them to try to determine the differences. Dr. J. Winkelman noted several features of the two disorders that were similar, but he gave one important factor that make these disorders different. In his article Sleep-Related Eating Disorder and Night Eating Syndrome: Sleep Disorders, Eating Disorders, Or both, Dr. Winkelman said, "Both [disorders] involve nearly nightly binging at multiple nocturnal awakenings, defined as excess calorie intake or loss of control over consumption." He also reported that both disorders have a common occurrence of approximately one to five percent of adults, have been predominantly found in women, with a young adult onset, have a chronic course, have a primary morbidity of weight gain, sleep disruption, and shame over loss of control over food intake, have familial bases, and have been observed to have comorbid depression and daytime eating disorders. However, Winkelman said, "The most prominent cited distinction between NES and SRED is the level of consciousness during nighttime eating episodes." Therefore, these two disorders are extremely similar with only one distinction between them. This information provided by Dr. Winkelman shows how doctors and psychologists have difficulty differentiating between NES and NSRED, but the distinction of a person's level of consciousness is what doctors chiefly rely on to make a diagnosis. One mistake that is often made is the misdiagnosis of NSRED for NES. However, even though NSRED is not a commonly known and diagnosed disease, many people suffer from it in differing ways while doctors work to find a treatment that works for everyone; several studies have been done on NSRED, such as the one conducted by Schenk and Mahowald. These studies, in turn, provide the basic information on this disorder including the symptoms, behaviors, and possible treatments that doctors are using today.

Signs and symptoms

Over the past thirty years, several studies have found that those afflicted with NSRED all have different symptoms and behaviors specific to them, yet they also all have similar characteristics that doctors and psychologists have identified to distinguish NSRED from other combinations of sleep and eating disorders such as Night Eating Syndrome. Dr. John W. Winkelman says that typical behaviors for patients with NSRED include: "Partial arousals from sleep, usually within 2 to 3 hours of sleep onset, and subsequent ingestion of food in a rapid or 'out of control' manner." They also will attempt to eat bizarre amalgamations of foods and even potentially harmful substances such as glue, wood, or other toxic materials. In addition, Schenck and Mahowald noted that their patients mainly ate sweets, pastas, both hot and cold meals, improper substances such as "raw, frozen, or spoiled foods; salt or sugar sandwiches; buttered cigarettes; and odd mixtures prepared in a blender."

During the handling of this food, patients with NSRED distinguish themselves, as they are usually messy or harmful to themselves. Some eat their food with their bare hands while others attempt to eat it with utensils. This occasionally results in injuries to the person as well as other injuries. After completing their studies, Schenck and Mahowald said, "Injuries resulted from the careless cutting of food or opening of cans; consumption of scalding fluids (coffee) or solids (hot oatmeal); and frenzied running into walls, kitchen counters, and furniture." A few of the more notable symptoms of this disorder include large amounts of weight gain over short periods of time, particularly in women; irritability during the day, due to lack of restful sleep; and vivid dreams at night. It is easily distinguished from regular sleepwalking by the typical behavioral sequence consisting of "rapid, 'automatic' arising from bed, and immediate entry into the kitchen." In addition, throughout all of the studies done, doctors and psychiatrists discovered that these symptoms are invariant across weekdays, weekends, and vacations as well as the eating excursions being erratically spread throughout a sleep cycle. Most people that suffer from this disease retain no control over when they arise and consume food in their sleep. Although some have been able to restrain themselves from indulging in their unconscious appetites, some have not and must turn to alternative methods of stopping this disorder. It is important for trained physicians to recognize these symptoms in their patients as quickly as possible, so those with NSRED may be treated before they injure themselves.

Treatment

For those patients who have not been able to stop this disorder on their own, doctors have been working to discover a treatment that will work for everyone. One treatment that Schenck and Mahowald studied consisted of psychotherapy combined with "environmental manipulation." This was usually done separately from the weight-reducing diets. However, during this study only 10 percent of the patients were able to lose more than one third of their initial excess weight, which was not a viable percentage. In addition, they reported that many of the patients experienced "major depression" and "severe anxiety" during the attempted treatments. This was not one of the most successful attempts to help those with NSRED.

However, Dr. R. Auger reported on another trial treatment where patients were treated utilizing pramipexole. Those conducting the treatment noticed how the nocturnal median motor activity was decreased, as was assessed by actigraphy, and individual progress of sleep quality was reported. Nevertheless, Dr. Augur also said, "27 percent of subjects had RLS (Restless Legs Syndrome, a condition known to respond to this medication), and number and duration of waking episodes related to eating behaviors were unchanged." (Bad link to this source. Please pro ide proper source.) Encouraged by the positive response verified in the above-mentioned trial treatment, doctors and psychiatrists conducted a more recent study described by Dr. Auger as "efficacy of topiramate [an antiepileptic drug associated with weight loss] in 17 consecutive patients with NSRED." Out of the 65 percent of patients who continued to take the medication on a regular basis, all confirmed either considerable development or absolute remission of "night-eating" in addition to "significant weight loss" being achieved. (Bad link to this source. Please provide proper source.) This has been one of the most effective treatments discovered so far, but many patients still suffered from NSRED. Therefore, other treatments were sought after.

Such treatments include those targeted to associated sleep disorders with the hope that it would play an essential part of the treatment process of NSRED. In Schenck and Mahowald's series, combinations of cardibopa/L-dopa, codeine, and clonazepam were used to treat five patients with RLS and one patient with somnambulism and PLMS (Periodic Limb Movements in Sleep). These patients all were suffering from NSRED as well as these other disorders, and they all experienced a remission of their NSRED as a result of taking these drugs. Two patients with OSA (Obstructive Sleep Apnea) and NSRED also reported as having a "resolution of their symptoms with nasal continuous positive airway pressure (nCPAP) therapy." Clonazepam monotherapy was also found to be successful in 50 percent of patients with simultaneous somnambulism. Interestingly, dopaminergic agents such as monotherapy were effective in 25 percent of the NSRED subgroup. Success with combinations of dopaminergic and opioid drugs, with the occasional addition of sedatives, also was found in seven patients without associated sleep disorders. In those for whom opioids and sedatives are relatively contraindicated (e.g., in those with histories of substance abuse), two case reports were described as meeting with success with a combination of bupropion, levodopa, and trazodone. Notably, hypnotherapy, psychotherapy, and various behavioral techniques, including environmental manipulation, were not effective on the majority of the patients studied. Nevertheless, Dr. Auger argue that behavioral strategies should complement the overall treatment plan and should include deliberate placement of food to avoid indiscriminate wandering, maintenance of a safe sleep environment, and education regarding proper sleep hygiene and stress management. (Bad link to source. Please provideproper source.) Even with their extensive studies, Schenck and Mahowald did not find the success as Dr. Auger found by treating his patients with topiramate.

History

The first case of NSRED was reported in 1955, but over the next thirty-six years, only nine more reports were made of this syndrome. Seven of these reports were single-case studies and the other two instances were seen during objective sleep studies, all done by psychiatrists and doctors. Schenck and Mahowald were the first to a major study on this disorder. They started their study of NSRED in 1985 and continued until 1993 with several cases among a total of 38 other various sleep-related disorders. Many of the cases they observed had symptoms that overlapped with those of NES, but this study was the first to discover that NSRED was different from NES in the fact that those suffering from NSRED were either partially or completely unaware of their actions at night while those with NES were aware. Schenck and Mahowald also discovered that none of the patients had any eating instability before their problems at night while sleeping. In their 1993 report, they summarized the major findings with the idea that women encompass at least two thirds of the patients and that the majority of these patients had become overweight. They also discovered that while the patients' night-eating normally started during early adulthood, this wasn't always the case as it started as early as childhood to as late as middle adulthood. These patients not only had NSRED, but many of them had also been suffering from other nighttime behaviors such as sleep terrors for several years. This revolutionized the way people saw NSRED. With the technological age growing and more people becoming obese, Schenck and Mahowald's discovery of NSRED causing a large weight increase helped doctors more easily identify this disorder. Almost half of Schenck and Mahowald's patients were significantly obese. According to body mass index's criteria, no patient was emaciated. Schenck and Mahowald said, "virtually all patients had accurate non-distorted appraisals of their body size, shape, and weight. Furthermore, unlike the patients in Stunkard's series, none of our patients had problematic eating in the evening between dinner and bedtime; sleep onset insomnia was not present; and sleep latency was usually brief, apart from several patients with RLS." After realizing what was wrong with them, many of Schenck and Mahowald's patients with NSRED restricted their day eating and over exercised. It identifies the first initial findings concerning NSRED, and it shows how NSRED is a random malady that affects many different types of people in individual ways.

Rumination Syndrome

Rumination syndrome, or Merycism, is an under-diagnosed chronic motility disorder characterized by effortless regurgitation of most meals following consumption, due to the involuntary contraction of the muscles around the abdomen. There is no retching, nausea, heartburn, odour, or abdominal pain associated with the regurgitation, as there is with typical vomiting. The disorder has been historically documented as affecting only infants, young children, and people with cognitive disabilities (the prevalence is as high as 10% in institutionalized patients with various mental disabilities). Today it is being diagnosed in increasing numbers of otherwise healthy adolescents and adults, though there is a lack of awareness of the condition by doctors, patients and the general public.

Rumination syndrome presents itself in a variety of ways, with especially high contrast existing between the presentation of the typical adult sufferer without a mental disability and the presentation of an infant and/or mentally impaired sufferer. Like related gastrointestinal disorders, rumination can adversely affect normal functioning and the social lives of individuals. It has been linked with depression.

Little comprehensive data regarding rumination syndrome in otherwise healthy individuals exists because most sufferers are private about their illness and are often misdiagnosed due to the number of symptoms and the clinical similarities between rumination syndrome and other disorders of the stomach and esophagus, such as gastroparesis and bulimia nervosa. These symptoms include the acid-induced erosion of the esophagus and enamel, halitosis, malnutrition, severe weight loss and an unquenchable appetite. Individuals may begin regurgitating within a minute following ingestion, and the full cycle of ingestion and regurgitation can mimic the binging and purging of bulimia.

Diagnosis of rumination syndrome is non-invasive and based on a history of the individual. Treatment is promising, with upwards of 85% of individuals responding positively to treatment, including infants and the mentally handicapped.

Classification

Rumination syndrome is a condition which affects the functioning of the stomach and esophagus, also known as a *functional gastroduodenal disorder*. In patients that have a history of eating disorders, Rumination syndrome is grouped alongside eating disorders such as bulimia and pica, which are themselves grouped under non-psychotic mental disorder. In most healthy adolescents and adults who have no mental disability, Rumination syndrome is considered a motility disorder instead of an eating disorder, because the patients tend to have had no control over its occurrence and have had no history of eating disorders.

Signs and Symptoms

While the number and severity of symptoms varies among individuals, repetitive regurgitation of undigested food (known as rumination) after the start of a meal is always present. In some individuals, the regurgitation is small, occurring over a long period of time following ingestion, and can be rechewed and swallowed. In others, the amount can be bilious and short lasting, and must be expelled. While some only experience symptoms following some meals, most experience episodes following any ingestion, from a single bite to a massive feast. However, some long-term patients will find a select couple of food or drink items that do not trigger a response.

Unlike typical vomiting, the regurgitation is typically described as effortless and unforced. There is seldom nausea preceding the expulsion, and the undigested food lacks the bitter taste and odour of stomach acid and bile.

Symptoms can begin to manifest at any point from the ingestion of the meal to 120 minutes thereafter. However, the more common range is between 30 seconds to 1 hour after the completion of a meal. Symptoms tend to cease when the ruminated contents become acidic.

Abdominal pain (38.1%), lack of fecal production or constipation (21.1%), nausea (17.0%), diarrhea (8.2%), bloating (4.1%), and dental decay (3.4%) are also described as common symptoms in day-to-day life. These symptoms are not necessarily prevalent during regurgitation episodes, and can happen at any time. Weight loss is often observed (42.2%) at an average loss of 9.6 kilograms, and is more common in cases where the disorder has gone undiagnosed for a longer period of time, though this may be expected of the nutrition deficiencies that often accompany the disorder as a consequence of its symptoms. Depression has also been linked with rumination syndrome, though its effects on rumination syndrome are unknown.

Acid erosion of the teeth can be a feature of rumination, as can halitosis (bad breath).

Causes

The cause of rumination syndrome is unknown. However, studies have drawn a correlation between hypothesized causes and the history of patients with the disorder. In infants and the cognitively impaired, the disease has normally been attributed to over-stimulation and under-stimulation from parents and caregivers, causing the individual to seek self-gratification and self-stimulus due to the lack or abundance of external stimuli. The disorder has also commonly been attributed to a bout of illness, a period of stress in the individual's recent past, and to changes in medication.

In adults and adolescents, hypothesized causes generally fall into one of either category: habit-induced, and trauma-induced. Habit-induced individuals generally have a history of bulimia nervosa or of intentional regurgitation (magicians and professional regurgitators, for example), which though initially self-induced, forms a subconscious habit that can continue to manifest itself outside the control of the affected individual. Trauma-induced individuals describe an emotional or physical injury (such as recent surgery, psychological distress, concussions, deaths in the family, etc.), which preceded the onset of rumination, often by several months.

Diagnosis

Rumination syndrome is diagnosed based on a complete history of the individual. Costly and invasive studies such as gastroduodenal manometry and esophageal Ph testing are unnecessary and will often aid in misdiagnosis. Based on typical observed features, several criteria have been suggested for diagnosing rumination syndrome. The primary symptom, the regurgitation of recently ingested food, must be consistent, occurring for at least six weeks of the past twelve months. The regurgitation must begin within 30 minutes of the completion of a meal. Patients may either chew the regurgitated matter or expel it. The symptoms must stop within 90 minutes, or when the regurgitated matter becomes acidic. The symptoms must not be the result of a mechanical obstruction, and should not respond to the standard treatment for gastroesophageal reflux disease.

In adults, the diagnosis is supported by the absence of classical or structural diseases of the gastrointestinal system. Supportive criteria include a regurgitant that does not taste sour or acidic, is generally odourless, is effortless, or at most preceded by a belching sensation, that there is no retching preceding the regurgitation, and that the act is not associated with nausea or heartburn.

Patients visit an average of five physicians over 2.75 years before being correctly diagnosed with rumination syndrome.

Differential Diagnosis

Rumination syndrome in adults is a complicated disorder whose symptoms can mimic those of several other gastroesophogeal disorders and diseases. Bulimia nervosa and gastroparesis are especially prevalent among the misdiagnoses of rumination.

Bulimia nervosa, among adults and especially adolescents, is by far the most common misdiagnosis patients will hear during their experiences with rumination syndrome. This is due to the similarities in symptoms to an outside observer—"vomiting" following food intake—which, in long-term patients, may include ingesting copious amounts to offset malnutrition, and a lack of willingness to expose their condition and its symptoms. While it has been suggested that there is a connection between rumination and bulimia, unlike bulimia, rumination is not self-inflicted. Adults and adolescents with rumination syndrome are generally well aware of their gradually increasing malnutrition, but are unable to control the reflex. In contrast, those with bulimia intentionally induce vomiting, and seldom re-swallow food.

Gastroparesis is another common misdiagnosis. Like rumination syndrome, patients with gastroparesis often bring up food following the ingestion of a meal. Unlike rumination, gastroparesis causes vomiting (in contrast to regurgitation) of food, which is not being digested further, from the stomach. This vomiting occurs several hours after a meal is ingested, preceded by nausea and retching, and has the bitter or sour taste typical of vomit.

Pathophysiology

Rumination syndrome is a poorly understood disorder, and a number of theories have speculated the mechanisms that cause the regurgitation, which is a unique symptom to this disorder. While no theory has gained a consensus, some are more notable and widely published than others.

The most widely documented mechanism is that the ingestion of food causes gastric distention, which is followed by abdominal compression and the simultaneous relaxation of the lower esophageal sphincter (LES). This creates a common cavity between the stomach and the oropharynx that allows the partially digested material to return to the mouth. There are several offered explanations for the sudden relaxation of the LES. Among these explanations is that it is a learned voluntary relaxation, which is common in those with or having had bulimia. While this relaxation may be voluntary, the overall process of rumination is still generally involuntary. Relaxation due to intra-abdominal pressure is another proposed explanation, which would make abdominal compression the primary mechanism. The third is an adaptation of the belch reflex, which is the most commonly described mechanism. The swallowing of air immediately prior to regurgitation causes the activation of the belching reflex that triggers the relaxation of the LES. Patients often describe a feeling similar to the onset of a belch preceding rumination.

Treatment and Prognosis

There is presently no known cure for rumination. Proton pump inhibitors and other medications have been used to little or no effect. Treatment is different for infants and the mentally handicapped than for adults and adolescents of normal intelligence. For adults and adolescents,Biofeedback and relaxation techniques, to be practice after eating or whenever regurgitation occurs, has proven to be most effective. Among infants and the mentally handicapped, behavioral and mild aversive training has been shown to cause improvement in most cases. Aversive training involves associating the ruminating behavior with negative results, and rewarding good behavior and eating. Placing a sour or bitter taste on the tongue when the individual begins the movements or breathing patterns typical of his or her ruminating behavior is the generally accepted method for aversive training, although some older studies advocate the use of pinching. In patients of normal intelligence, rumination is not an intentional behavior and is habitually reversed using diaphragmatic breathing to counter the urge to regurgitate. Alongside reassurance, explanation and habit reversal, patients are shown how to breathe using their diaphragms prior to and during the normal rumination period. A similar breathing pattern can be used to prevent normal vomiting. Breathing in this method works by physically preventing the abdominal contractions required to expel stomach contents.

Supportive therapy and diaphragmatic breathing has shown to cause improvement in 56% of cases, and total cessation of symptoms in an additional 30% in one study of 54 adolescent patients who were followed up 10 months after initial treatments. Patients who successfully use the technique often notice an immediate change in health for the better. Individuals who have had bulimia or who intentionally induced vomiting in the past have a reduced chance for improvement due to the reinforced behavior. The technique is not used with infants or young children due to the complex timing and concentration required for it to be successful. Most infants grow out of the disorder within a year or with aversive training.

Epidemiology

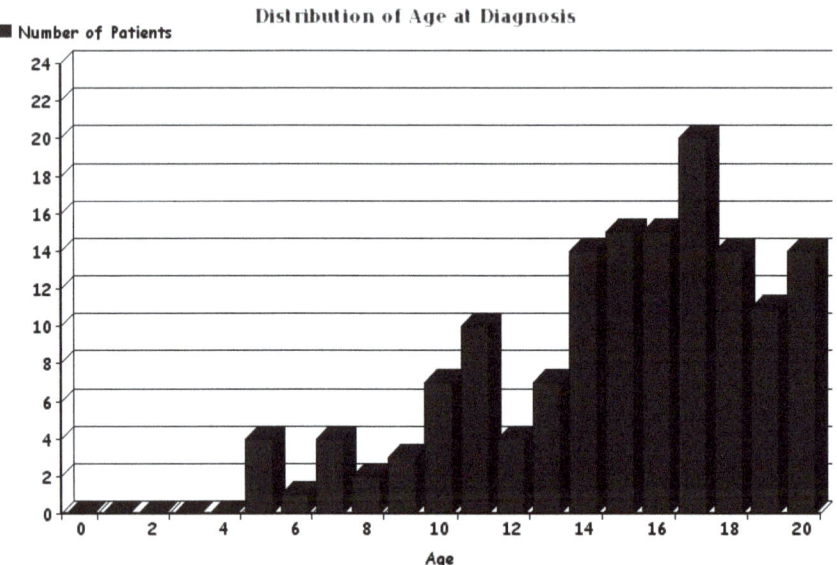

Age distribution at diagnosis

Rumination disorder was initially documented as affecting newborns, infants, children and individuals with mental and functional disabilities (the cognitively handicapped). It has since been recognized to occur in both males and females of all ages and cognitive abilities.

Among the latter, it is described with almost equal prevalence among infants (6–10% of the population) and institutionalized adults (8–10%). In infants, it typically occurs within the first 3–12 months of age.

The occurrence of rumination syndrome within the general population has not been defined. Rumination is sometimes described as rare, but has also been described as not rare, but rather rarely recognized. The disorder has a female predominance. The typical age of adolescent onset is 12.9, give or take 0.4 years (±), with males affected sooner than females (11.0 ± 0.8 for males versus 13.8 ± 0.5 for females).

There is little evidence concerning the impact of hereditary influence in rumination syndrome. However, case reports involving entire families with rumination exist.

History

The term *rumination* is derived from the Latin word *ruminare*, which means *to chew the cud*. First described in ancient times, and mentioned in the writings of Aristotle, rumination syndrome was clinically documented in 1618 by Italian anatomist Fabricus ab Aquapendende, who wrote of the symptoms in a patient of his.

Among the earliest cases of rumination was that of a physician in the nineteenth century, Charles-Édouard Brown-Séquard, who acquired the condition as the result of experiments upon himself. As a way of evaluating and testing the acid response of the stomach to various foods, the doctor would swallow sponges tied to a string, then intentionally regurgitate them to analyze the contents. As a result of these experiments, the doctor eventually regurgitated his meals habitually by reflex.

Numerous case reports exist from before the twentieth century, but were influenced greatly by the methods and thinking used in that time. By the early twentieth century, it was becoming increasingly evident that rumination presented itself in a variety of ways in response to a variety of conditions. Although still considered a disorder of infancy and cognitive disability at that time, the difference in presentation between infants and adults was well established.

Studies of rumination in otherwise healthy adults became decreasingly rare starting in the 1900s, and the majority of published reports analyzing the syndrome in mentally healthy patients appeared thereafter. At first, adult rumination was described and treated as a benign condition. It is now described as otherwise. While the base of patients to examine has gradually increased as more and more people come forward with their symptoms, awareness of the condition by the medical community and the general public is still limited.

In other Animals

The chewing of cud by animals such as cows, goats, and giraffes is considered normal behavior. These animals are known as ruminants. Such behavior, though termed rumination, is not related to human rumination syndrome, but is ordinary. Involuntary rumination, similar to what is seen in humans, has been described in gorillas and other primates.

Purging Disorder

Purging disorder is an eating disorder characterized by recurrent purging (self-induced vomiting, misuse of laxatives, diuretics, or enemas) to control weight or shape in the absence of binge eating episodes that occurs in people with normal or near-normal weight. Purging disorder differs from anorexia nervosa (AN) because individuals with purging disorder are not underweight, and Purging disorder differs from bulimia nervosa (BN) because individuals with purging disorder do not consume a large amount of food before they purge. In current diagnostic systems, purging disorder is a form of Other specified feeding or eating disorder (OSFED). Research indicates that purging disorder may be as common as bulimia nervosa or anorexia nervosa in women, that the syndrome is associated with clinically significant levels of distress, and that it appears to be distinct from bulimia nervosa on measures of hunger and ability to control food intake. Some of the signs of purging disorder are frequent trips to the bathroom directly after a meal, frequent use of laxatives, and obsession over one's appearance and weight. Other signs include swollen cheeks, popped blood vessels in the eyes, and clear teeth which are all signs of excessive vomiting.

References

- Hay, P (July 2013). "A systematic review of evidence for psychological treatments in eating disorders: 2005–2012.". The International Journal of Eating Disorders. 46 (5): 462–9. PMID 23658093. doi:10.1002/eat.22103

- Diagnostic and statistical manual of mental disorders : DSM-5 (5 ed.). Washington: American Psychiatric Publishing. 2013. pp. 338–345. ISBN 978-0-89042-555-8

- "Eating Disorders Anorexia Causes | Eating Disorders". Psychiatric Disorders and Mental Health Issues. Retrieved 1 March 2016

- Attia E (2010). "Anorexia Nervosa: Current Status and Future Directions". Annual Review of Medicine. 61 (1): 425–35. PMID 19719398. doi:10.1146/annurev.med.050208.200745

- Haller E (1992). "Eating disorders. A review and update". The Western Journal of Medicine. 157 (6): 658–62. PMC 1022101. PMID 1475950

- Robinson, Paul H. (2006). Community treatment of eating disorders. Chichester: John Wiley & Sons. p. 66. ISBN 978-0-470-01676-3

- "An update of 'The Neglected Crisis of Undernutrition: Evidence for Action'" (PDF). www.gov.uk. Department for International Development. Oct 2012. Retrieved 5 July 2014

- Halmi KA (2013). "Perplexities of treatment resistance in eating disorders". BMC Psychiatry. 13: 292. PMC 3829659. PMID 24199597. doi:10.1186/1471-244X-13-292

- Misra, Madhusmita; Klibanski, Anne (1 June 2014). "Anorexia nervosa and bone". Journal of Endocrinology. 221 (3): R163–R176. ISSN 0022-0795. PMC 4047520. PMID 24898127. doi:10.1530/JOE-14-0039

- Kleinman R (1 April 2008). Walker's Pediatric Gastrointestinal Disease. PMPH-USA. ISBN 978-1-55009-364-3. Retrieved 9 April 2015

- "Global hunger declining, but still unacceptably high International hunger targets difficult to reach" (PDF). Food and Agriculture Organization of the United Nations. September 2010. Retrieved 1 July 2014

- Lozano GA (2008). "Obesity and sexually selected anorexia nervosa". Medical Hypotheses. 71 (6): 933–940. PMID 18760541. doi:10.1016/j.mehy.2008.07.013

- J. C. Waterlow (1972). "Classification and Definition of Protein-Calorie Malnutrition". British Medical Journal. 3 (5826): 566–569. PMC 1785878. PMID 4627051. doi:10.1136/bmj.3.5826.566

- Malthus, Thomas Robert; Appleman, Philip (1976). An essay on the principle of population: text, sources and background, criticism. Norton. ISBN 978-0-393-09202-8

- Alina Paul Bossuet, Nourishing Communities Through Holistic Farming "Archived copy". Archived from the original on April 2, 2015. Retrieved 2014-01-26. . ICRISAT. Downloaded 26 January 2014

- Gowers S. G.; et al. (2000). "Impact of hospitalisation on the outcome of adolescent anorexia nervosa". Br J Psychiatry. 176 (2): 138–141. doi:10.1192/bjp.176.2.138

- Hay, P (July 2013). "A systematic review of evidence for psychological treatments in eating disorders: 2005–2012.". The International Journal of Eating Disorders. 46 (5): 462–9. PMID 23658093. doi:10.1002/eat.22103

- Wang, Youfa (2012). Capter 2. Use of Percentiles and Z-Scores in Anthropometry. In Handbook of Anthropometry. New York: Springer. p. 29. ISBN 978-1-4419-1787-4

- "Obesity Education Initiative Electronic Textbook - Treatment Guidelines". US National Institutes of Health. Retrieved 29 July 2016

- Vyver E, Steinegger C, Katzman DK (2008). "Eating disorders and menstrual dysfunction in adolescents". Ann. N. Y. Acad. Sci. 1135: 253–64. PMID 18574232. doi:10.1196/annals.1429.013

- Campos, Paul (8 December 2005). "The epidemiology of overweight and obesity: public health crisis or moral health?". International Journal of Epidemiology

- Association], American Psychiatry (2013). Diagnostic and statistical manual of mental disorders: DSM-5 (5th ed.). Washington [etc.]: American Psychiatric Publishing. p. 350. ISBN 0890425558

- Douglas Harper (November 2001). "Online Etymology Dictionary: bulimia". Online Etymology Dictionary. Retrieved 2008-04-06

- Kastin DA, Buchman AL (2002). "Malnutrition and gastrointestinal disease.". Curr Opin Clin Nutr Metab Care (Review). 5 (6): 699–706. PMID 12394647. doi:10.1097/01.mco.0000038815.16540.bc

- Saguy, Abigail; Gruys, Kiersten. "Morality and Health: News Media Constructions of Overweight and Eating Disorders" (PDF). UCLA. Retrieved Nov 2014

- Wynn DR, Martin MJ; Martin (1984). "A physical sign of bulimia". Mayo Clinic Proceedings. 59 (10): 722. PMID 6592415. doi:10.1016/s0025-6196(12)62063-1

3

Eating Disorder: Diagnostic Techniques

Eating disorders can be diagnosed by using several diagnostic techniques like eating attitudes test, eating disorder inventory, SCOFF questionnaire, body attitudes questionnaire, body mass index, etc. Only a trained professional can take these tests. The aspects elucidated in this chapter are of vital importance, and provide a better understanding of eating disorders.

Eating Attitudes Test

The Eating Attitudes Test (EAT, EAT-26), created by David Garner, is a widely used self-report questionnaire 26-item standardized self-report measure of symptoms and concerns characteristic of eating disorders. The EAT has been a particularly useful screening tool to assess "eating disorder risk" in high school, college and other special risk samples such as athletes. Screening for eating disorders is based on the assumption that early identification can lead to earlier treatment, thereby reducing serious physical and psychological complications or even death. Furthermore, EAT has been extremely effective in screening for anorexia nervosa in many populations.

The EAT-26 can be used in a non-clinical as well as a clinical setting not specifically focused on eating disorders. It can be administered in group or individual settings and is designed to be administered by mental health professionals, school counselors, coaches, camp counselors, and others with interest in gathering information to determine if an individual should be referred to a specialist for evaluation for an eating disorder. It is ideally suited for school settings, athletic programs, fitness centers, infertility clinics, pediatric practices, general practice settings, and outpatient psychiatric departments. It is designed for adolescents and adults.

The EAT-26 is rated on a six-point scale based on how often the individual engages in specific behaviors. The questions may be answered: Always, Usually, Often, Sometimes, Rarely, and Never. Completing the EAT-26 yields a "referral index" based on three criteria: 1) the total score based on the answers to the EAT-26 questions; 2) answers to the behavioral questions related to eating symptoms and weight loss, and 3) the individual's body mass index (BMI) calculated from their height and weight. Generally a referral is recommended if a respondent scores "positively" or meets the "cut off" scores or threshold on one or more criteria.

Development and History

The EAT was developed in response to a National Institute of Mental Health consensus panel that recognized a need for screening large populations to increase early identification of anorexia related symptoms. Additionally, the NIMH wanted a measure that could be used to examine the social and cultural factors involved in the development and maintenance of eating disorders The original version of the EAT was published in 1979, with 40 items each rated on a 6-point likert scale. In

1982, Garner and colleagues modified the original version to create an abbreviated 26-item test. The items were reduced after a factor analysis on the original 40-item data set revealed there to be only 26 independent items. Since that time, the EAT has been translated into many different languages and has gained widespread international as a tool to screen for eating disorders. Both the original paper and the subsequent 1982 publication are 3rd and 4th on the list of the 10 most cited articles in the history of the journal Psychological Medicine , a prominent peer-reviewed journal in the fields of psychology and psychiatry.

The EAT-26 should be used as the first step in a two-stage screening process. Accordingly, individuals who score higher than a 20 should be referred to a qualified professional to determine if they meet the diagnostic criteria for an eating disorder. The EAT-26 is not designed to make a diagnosis of an eating disorder and should not be used in place of a professional diagnosis or consultation. The EAT should only be used as a screener for general eating disorders, as research has not shown it to be a valid instrument in making specific diagnoses.

Permission to use the EAT-40 or EAT-26 can be obtained from David Garner through the EAT-26 website or the River Centre Clinic . Instructions and scoring information can be obtained from the EAT-26 website for no charge.

Limitations

The EAT suffers from the same problems as other self-report inventories, in that scores can be easily exaggerated or minimized by the person completing them. Like all questionnaires, the way the instrument is administered can have an effect on the final score. If a patient is asked to fill out the form in front of other people in a clinical environment, for instance, social expectations have been shown to elicit a different response compared to administration via a postal survey.

There are some general concerns with the EAT-26. First, varied symptoms of eating disorders and self-report instruments like the EAT measure symptoms only at that particular point in time. Therefore, considerable fluctuation is possible in some aspects of the eating disorder. Additionally, as it occurs with self-report measures generally, high scores on the EAT is typically influenced by a person's attitude. For example, a person might disclose less about their problems in order to be more socially desirable. The EAT has low positive predictive value because of denial and social desirability, as well as the possible confounding role of co-morbid factors.

Eating Disorder Inventory

The Eating Disorder Inventory (EDI) is a self-report questionnaire used to assess the presence of eating disorders, (a) Anorexia Nervosa both restricting and binge-eating/purging type; (b) Bulimia Nervosa; and (c) Eating disorder not otherwise specified including Binge Eating Disorder (BED). The original questionnaire consisted of 64 questions, divided into eight subscales.It was created in 1984 by David M. Garner et al. There have been two subsequent revisions by Garner; Eating disorder inventory-two (EDI-2) and Eating disorder inventory-three (EDI-3), published by Psychological Assessment Resources, Inc. located in Lutz, Florida.

Diagnostic use

The Eating disorder inventory is a diagnostic tool designed for use in a clinical setting to assess the presence of an eating disorder. Due to high comorbity associated with eating disorders it is generally used in conjunction with other psychological tests such as the Beck Depression Inventory. Depression has been shown to yield higher scores on the EDI-3.

EDI

The Eating disorder inventory (EDI) comprises 64 questions, divided into eight subscales. Each question is on a 6-point scale (ranging from 'always' to 'never'), rated 0-3. The score for each subscale is then summed. The 8 subscale scores on the EDI are:

1. Drive for thinness (DT): an excessive concern with dieting, preoccupation with weight, and fear of weight gain.

2. Bulimia: episodes of binge eating and purging

3. Body dissatisfaction: not being satisfied with one's physical appearance

4. Ineffectiveness: assesses feelings of inadequacy, insecurity, worthlessness and having no control over their lives.

5. Perfectionism:not being satisfied with anything less than perfect

6. Interpersonal distrust: reluctance to form close relationships

7. Interoceptive awareness (IA):"measures the ability of an individual to discriminate between sensations and feelings, and between the sensations of hunger and satiety",

8. Maturity fears:the fear of facing the demands of adult life

EDI-2

The first revision to the Eating disorder inventory was in 1991. The 1991 version, Eating disorder inventory-two (EDI-2) is used for both males and females over age 12. The EDI-2 retains the original format of the EDI with the inclusion of 27 new items divided into three additional subscales:

1. Asceticism:reflects the avoidance of sexual relationships

2. Impulse Regulation:shows the ability to regulate impulsive behavior, especially the binge behaviour

3. Social Insecurity: estimates social fears and insecurity

EDI-3

The latest revision to the Eating disorder inventory; Eating disorder inventory-three (EDI-3) was released in 2004. It contains the original items of the first EDI as well as EDI-2, it has been enhanced to reflect more modern theories related to the diagnosis of eating disorders. It was designed for use with females ages 13–53 years. It contains 91 items divided into twelve subscales rated on a 0-4 point scoring system. 3 items are specific to eating disorders and 9 are general psychological scales that while not specific are relevant to eating disorders. It yields six composites: Eating Disorder Risk, Ineffectiveness, Interpersonal Problems, Affective Problems, Overcontrol, General Psychological Maladjustment. It is also a self-report questionnaire administered in twenty minutes.

EDI-3SC

The Eating disorder symptom checklist (EDI-3SC) is a separate self-report form used to measure the frequency of symptoms, (i.e. binge eating; use of laxatives, diet pills; exercise patterns). The information provided by the EDI-3SC aids in determining whether the patient meets the diagnostic criteria as set forth in the Diagnostic and Statical Manual of Mental Disorders IV-TR (DSM-IV) for an eating disorder.

EDI-3RF

The Eating disorder referral form (EDI-3RF) is an abbreviated form of the EDI-3 for use in non-clinical settings for use in the allied health professions. It contains 25 questions from the EDI-3 from the three scales that are specific to eating disorder risk. It also includes questions specific to the behavioral patterns of someone with or at risk of developing an eating disorder. The EDI-3RF also utilizes referral indexes based on Body Mass Index (BMI) in identifying at risk patients

SCOFF Questionnaire

The SCOFF questionnaire utilizes an acronym in a simple five question test devised for use by non-professionals to assess the possible presence of an eating disorder. It was devised by Morgan *et al.* in 1999. The original SCOFF questionnaire was devised for use in the United Kingdom, thus the original acronym needs to be adjusted for users in the United States and Canada. The "S" in SCOFF stands for "Sick" which in British English means specifically to vomit. In American English and Canadian English it is synonymous with "ill". The "O" is used in the acronym to denote "one stone". A "stone" is an Imperial unit of weight which is equivalent to 6.35 kg. metric weight and 14 lbs. The letters in the full acronym are taken from key words in the questions:

- Sick
- Control
- One stone (14 lbs./6.5 kg.)
- Fat
- Food

Scoring

One point is assigned for every "yes"; a score greater than two (≥2) indicates a possible case of anorexia nervosa or bulimia nervosa.

Eating Disorder Examination Interview

The Eating Disorder Examination Interview (EDE) devised by Cooper & Fairburn (1987) is a semi-structured interview conducted by a clinician in the assessment of an eating disorder.

EDE

The EDE is a semi-structured interview conducted by a trained clinician to assess the psychopathology associated with the diagnosis of an eating disorder. The EDE is rated through the use of four subscales and a global score. The four subscales are:

1. Restraint

2. Eating concern

3. Shape concern

4. Weight concern

The questions concern the frequency in which the patient engages in behaviors indicative of an eating disorder over a 28-day period. The test is scored on a 7-point scale from 0-6. With a zero score indicating not having engaged in the questioned behavior.

EDE-Q

The Eating Disorders Examination Questionnaire (EDE-Q) was adapted from the EDE. The EDE-Q is a 41 item self-report questionnaire. It retains the format of the EDE including the 4 subscales and global score. It also concerns behaviors over a 28-day time period and retains the scoring system of 0-6, with 0 indicating no days, 1=1–5 days, 2=6–12 days, 3=13–15 days, 4=16–22 days, 5=23–27 days and 6= every day.

Body Attitudes Questionnaire

The Ben-Tovim Walker Body Attitudes Questionnaire (BAQ) is a 44 item self-report questionnaire divided into six subscales that measures a woman's attitude towards their own body. The BAQ is used in the assessment of eating disorders. It was devised by D.I. Ben-Tovim and M.K. Walker in 1991.

The six subscales measured by the BAQ are:

1.   Overall fatness

2.   Self disparagement

3.   Strength

4.   Salience of weight

5.   Feelings of attractiveness

6.   Consciousness of lower body fat

Foreign Language Versions

Portuguese Version

The BAQ was the first body attitudes scale to be translated into Portuguese. The validity of the Portuguese language version was proven in a test conducted on a cohort of Brazilian women who speak Portuguese as their native language. The test-retest reliability was .57 and .85 after a one-month interval. The test was conducted by Scagliusi *et al.*

Japanese Version

The BAQ was translated into Japanese and tested on 68 males and 139 females in Japan and 68 Japanese males living in Australia (Kagawa *et al.*) The scores were assessed against 72 Australian men using the English-language version as well as scores from previous female Australian participants. There was a significant difference between the Japanese and Australian groups (p,0.05). The BAQ was deemed adequate for use in both Japanese males and females.

Eating Disorder Diagnostic Scale

The Eating Disorder Diagnostic Scale (EDDS) is a 22 item self-report questionnaire that assesses the presence of three eating disorders; anorexia nervosa, bulimia nervosa and binge eating disorder. It was adapted by Stice *et al.* in 2000 from the validated structured psychiatric interview: The Eating Disorder Examination (EDE) and the eating disorder module of the Structured Clinical Interview for DSM-IV (SCID)16. In follow up studies of the reliability and validity of the EDDS it was shown to be sufficiently sensitive to detect the effects of eating disorders prevention programs, response to such programs and the future onset of eating disorder pathology and depression. The EDDS shows both full and subthreshold diagnoses for anorexia nervosa, bulimia nervosa and binge eating disorder. EDDS is a continuous eating disorder symptom composite score The PhenX Toolkit uses the EDDS for as an Eating Disorders Screener protocol.

Body Mass Index

The body mass index (BMI) or Quetelet index is a value derived from the mass (weight) and height of an individual. The BMI is defined as the body mass divided by the square of the body height, and is universally expressed in units of kg/m^2, resulting from mass in kilograms and height in metres.

The BMI may also be determined using a table or chart which displays BMI as a function of mass and height using contour lines or colours for different BMI categories, and which may use other units of measurement (converted to metric units for the calculation).

The BMI is an attempt to quantify the amount of tissue mass (muscle, fat, and bone) in an individual, and then categorize that person as *underweight, normal weight, overweight,* or *obese* based on that value. However, there is some debate about where on the BMI scale the dividing lines between categories should be placed. Commonly accepted BMI ranges are underweight: under 18.5 kg/m², normal weight: 18.5 to 25, overweight: 25 to 30, obese: over 30. People of Asian descent have different associations between BMI, percentage of body fat, and health risks than those of European descent, with a higher risk of type 2 diabetes and cardiovascular disease at BMIs lower than the WHO cut-off point for overweight, 25 kg/m², although the cutoff for observed risk varies among different Asian populations.

History

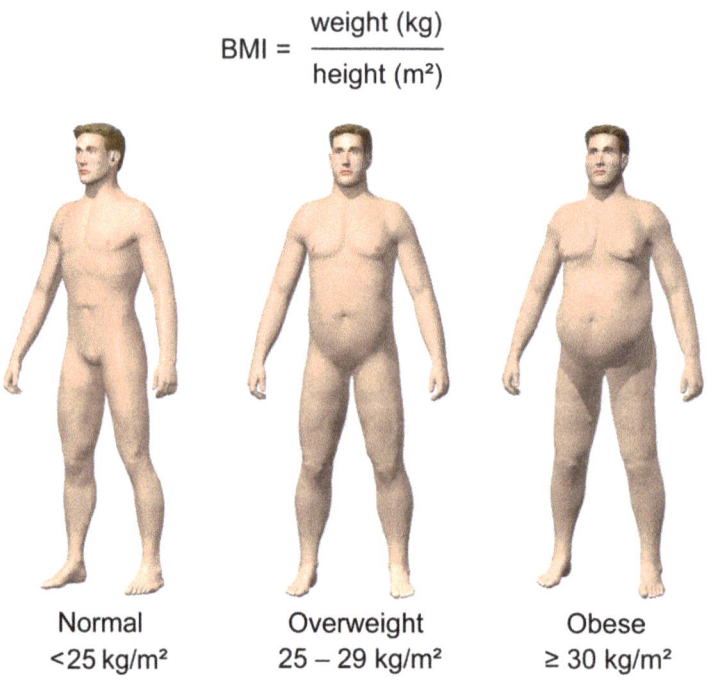

Obesity and Body Mass Index (BMI)

$$BMI = \frac{weight\ (kg)}{height\ (m^2)}$$

Normal
<25 kg/m²

Overweight
25 – 29 kg/m²

Obese
≥ 30 kg/m²

Obesity and BMI

The basis of the BMI was devised by Adolphe Quetelet, a Belgian astronomer, mathematician, statistician and sociologist, from 1830 to 1850 during which time he developed what he called "social physics". The modern term "body mass index" (BMI) for the ratio of human body weight to squared height was coined in a paper published in the July 1972 edition of the *Journal of Chronic Diseases* by Ancel Keys and others. In this paper, Keys argued that what he termed the BMI was "… if not fully satisfactory, at least as good as any other relative weight index as an indicator of relative obesity"

The interest in an index that measures body fat came with increasing obesity in prosperous Western societies. BMI was explicitly cited by Keys as appropriate for *population* studies and inappropriate for individual evaluation. Nevertheless, due to its simplicity, it has come to be widely used for preliminary diagnosis. Additional metrics, such as waist circumference, can be more useful.

The BMI is universally expressed in kg/m², resulting from mass in kilograms and height in metres. If pounds and inches are used, a conversion factor of 703 (kg/m²)/(lb/in²) must be applied. When the term BMI is used informally, the units are usually omitted.

BMI = mass kg height m 2 = mass lb height in 2 × 703

BMI provides a simple numeric measure of a person's *thickness* or *thinness*, allowing health professionals to discuss weight problems more objectively with their patients. BMI was designed to be used as a simple means of classifying average sedentary (physically inactive) populations, with an average body composition. For these individuals, the current value recommendations are as follow: a BMI from 18.5 up to 25 kg/m² may indicate optimal weight, a BMI lower than 18.5 suggests the person is underweight, a number from 25 up to 30 may indicate the person is overweight, and a number from 30 upwards suggests the person is obese. Some athletes, such as football linemen, have a high muscle to fat ratio and may have a BMI that is misleadingly high relative to their body fat percentage.

Scalability

BMI is proportional to the mass and inversely proportional to the square of the height. So, if all body dimensions double, and mass scales naturally with the cube of the height, then BMI doubles instead of remaining the same. This results in taller people having a reported BMI that is uncharacteristically high, compared to their actual body fat levels. In comparison, the Ponderal index is based on the natural scaling of mass with the third power of the height.

However, many taller people are not just "scaled up" short people but tend to have narrower frames in proportion to their height. Nick Korevaar (a mathematics lecturer from the University of Utah) suggests that instead of squaring the body height (as the BMI does) or cubing the body height (as the Ponderal index does), it would be more appropriate to use an exponent of between 2.3 and 2.7 (as originally noted by Quetelet). Carl Lavie has written that, "The B.M.I. tables are excellent for identifying obesity and body fat in large populations, but they are far less reliable for determining fatness in individuals."

Categories

A frequent use of the BMI is to assess how much an individual's body weight departs from what is normal or desirable for a person's height. The weight excess or deficiency may, in part, be accounted for by body fat (adipose tissue) although other factors such as muscularity also affect BMI significantly.

The WHO regards a BMI of less than 18.5 as underweight and may indicate malnutrition, an eating disorder, or other health problems, while a BMI equal to or greater than 25 is considered overweight and above 30 is considered obese. These ranges of BMI values are valid only as statistical categories.

Category	BMI (kg/m²)		BMI Prime	
	from	to	from	to
Very severely underweight		15		0.60
Severely underweight	15	16	0.60	0.64
Underweight	16	18.5	0.64	0.74
Normal (healthy weight)	18.5	25	0.74	1.0
Overweight	25	30	1.0	1.2
Obese Class I (Moderately obese)	30	35	1.2	1.4
Obese Class II (Severely obese)	35	40	1.4	1.6
Obese Class III (Very severely obese)	40		1.6	

BMI in Children (Aged 2 to 20)

BMI is used differently for children. It is calculated in the same way as for adults, but then compared to typical values for other children of the same age. Instead of comparison against fixed thresholds for underweight and overweight, the BMI is compared against the percentile for children of the same sex and age.

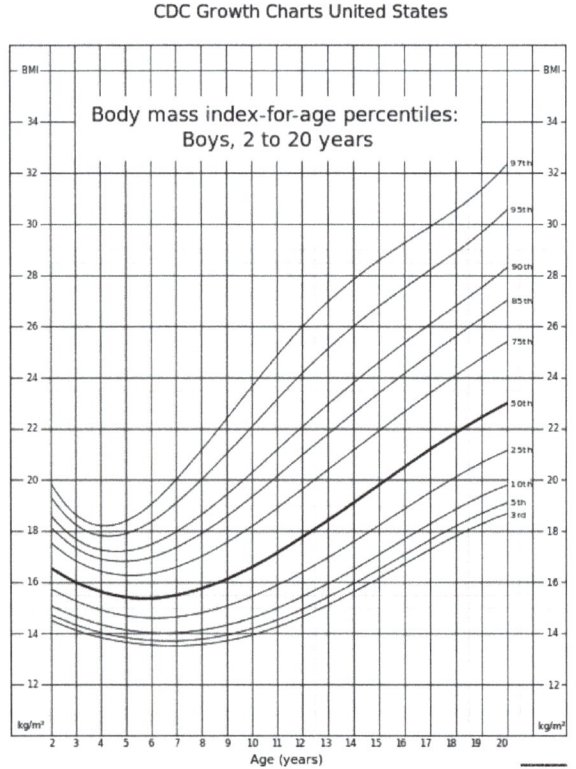

BMI for age percentiles for boys 2 to 20 years of age.

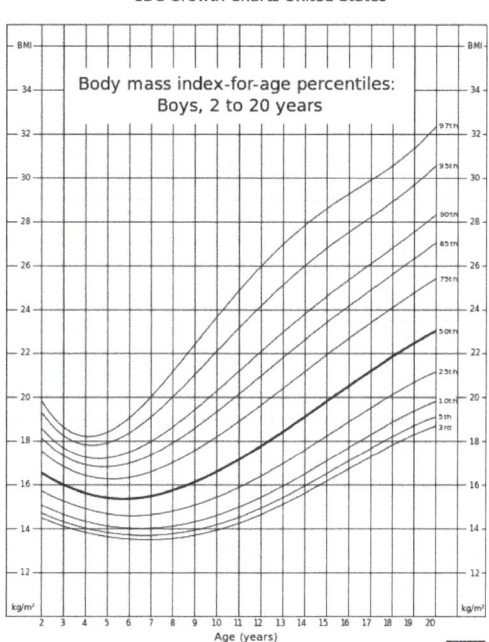

BMI for age percentiles for girls 2 to 20 years of age.

A BMI that is less than the 5th percentile is considered underweight and above the 95th percentile is considered obese. Children with a BMI between the 85th and 95th percentile are considered to be overweight.

Recent studies in Britain have indicated that females between the ages 12 and 16 have a higher BMI than males of the same age by 1.0 kg/m² on average.

International Variations

These recommended distinctions along the linear scale may vary from time to time and country to country, making global, longitudinal surveys problematic.

Hong Kong

The Hospital Authority of Hong Kong recommends the use of the following BMI ranges:

Category	BMI (kg/m²)	
	from	to
Underweight		18.5
Normal Range	18.5	23
Overweight—At Risk	23	25
Overweight—Moderately Obese	25	30
Overweight—Severely Obese	30	

Japan

Japan Society for the Study of Obesity (2000):

Category	BMI (kg/m²)	
	from	to
Low		18.5
Normal	18.5	25
Obese (Level 1)	25	30
Obese (Level 2)	30	35
Obese (Level 3)	35	40
Obese (Level 4)	40	

Singapore

In Singapore, the BMI cut-off figures were revised in 2005, motivated by studies showing that many Asian populations, including Singaporeans, have higher proportion of body fat and increased risk for cardiovascular diseases and diabetes mellitus, compared with Caucasians at the same BMI. The BMI cut-offs are presented with an emphasis on health risk rather than weight.

Health Risk	BMI (kg/m²)
Risk of developing problems such as nutritional deficiency and osteoporosis	under 18.5
Low Risk (healthy range)	18.5 to 23
Moderate risk of developing heart disease, high blood pressure, stroke, diabetes	23 to 27.5
High risk of developing heart disease, high blood pressure, stroke, diabetes	over 27.5

United States

In 1998, the U.S. National Institutes of Health and the Centers for Disease Control and Prevention brought U.S. definitions in line with World Health Organization guidelines, lowering the normal/ overweight cut-off from BMI 27.8 to BMI 25. This had the effect of redefining approximately 29 million Americans, previously *healthy*, to *overweight*.

This can partially explain the increase in the *overweight* diagnosis in the past 20 years, and the increase in sales of weight loss products during the same time. WHO also recommends lowering the normal/overweight threshold for South East Asian body types to around BMI 23, and expects further revisions to emerge from clinical studies of different body types.

The U.S. National Health and Nutrition Examination Survey of 1994 showed that 59.8% of American men and 51.2% of women had BMIs over 25. Morbid obesity—a BMI of 40 or more—was found in 2% of the men and 4% of the women. A survey in 2007 showed 63% of Americans are overweight or obese, with 26% in the obese category (a BMI of 30 or more). As of 2014, 37.7% of adults in the United States were obese, categorized as 35.0% of men and 40.4% of women; class 3 obesity (BMI over 40) values were 7.7% for men and 9.9% for women.

There are differing opinions on definition of underweight in females; doctors quote anything below 18.5 to 20 as underweight. The most frequently stated is 19. A BMI nearing 15 is usually defined as starvation and a BMI less than 17.5 as an informal criterion for the diagnosis of anorexia nervosa.

Body Mass Index values for males and females aged 20 and over, and selected percentiles by age: United States, 2011–2014.									
Age	Percentile								
	5th	10th	15th	25th	50th	75th	85th	90th	95th
	Men BMI (kg/m²)								
20 years and over (total)	20.7	22.2	23.0	24.6	27.7	31.6	34.0	36.1	39.8
20–29 years	19.3	20.5	21.2	22.5	25.5	30.5	33.1	35.1	39.2
30–39 years	21.1	22.4	23.3	24.8	27.5	31.9	35.1	36.5	39.3
40–49 years	21.9	23.4	24.3	25.7	28.5	31.9	34.4	36.5	40.0
50–59 years	21.6	22.7	23.6	25.4	28.3	32.0	34.0	35.2	40.3
60–69 years	21.6	22.7	23.6	25.3	28.0	32.4	35.3	36.9	41.2
70–79 years	21.5	23.2	23.9	25.4	27.8	30.9	33.1	34.9	38.9
80 years and over	20.0	21.5	22.5	24.1	26.3	29.0	31.1	32.3	33.8
Age	Women BMI (kg/m²)								
20 years and over (total)	19.6	21.0	22.0	23.6	27.7	33.2	36.5	39.3	43.3
20–29 years	18.6	19.8	20.7	21.9	25.6	31.8	36.0	38.9	42.0
30–39 years	19.8	21.1	22.0	23.3	27.6	33.1	36.6	40.0	44.7
40–49 years	20.0	21.5	22.5	23.7	28.1	33.4	37.0	39.6	44.5
50–59 years	19.9	21.5	22.2	24.5	28.6	34.4	38.3	40.7	45.2
60–69 years	20.0	21.7	23.0	24.5	28.9	33.4	36.1	38.7	41.8
70–79 years	20.5	22.1	22.9	24.6	28.3	33.4	36.5	39.1	42.9
80 years and over	19.3	20.4	21.3	23.3	26.1	29.7	30.9	32.8	35.2
Source: "Anthropometric Reference Data for Children and Adults: United States" from CDC DHHS									

Consequences of Elevated Level in Adults

The BMI ranges are based on the relationship between body weight and disease and death. Overweight and obese individuals are at an increased risk for the following diseases:

- Coronary artery disease

- Dyslipidemia

- Type 2 diabetes

- Gallbladder disease

- Hypertension

- Osteoarthritis

- Sleep apnea

- Stroke

- At least 10 cancers, including endometrial, breast, and colon cancer.

- Epidural lipomatosis

Among people who have never smoked, overweight/obesity is associated with 51% increase in mortality compared with people who have always been a normal weight.

Applications

Public Health

The BMI is generally used as a means of correlation between groups related by general mass and can serve as a vague means of estimating adiposity. The duality of the BMI is that, while it is easy to use as a general calculation, it is limited as to how accurate and pertinent the data obtained from it can be. Generally, the index is suitable for recognizing trends within sedentary or overweight individuals because there is a smaller margin of error. The BMI has been used by the WHO as the standard for recording obesity statistics since the early 1980s.

This general correlation is particularly useful for consensus data regarding obesity or various other conditions because it can be used to build a semi-accurate representation from which a solution can be stipulated, or the RDA for a group can be calculated. Similarly, this is becoming more and more pertinent to the growth of children, due to the fact that the majority of children are sedentary.

Clinical Practice

BMI categories are generally regarded as a satisfactory tool for measuring whether sedentary individuals are *underweight*, *overweight*, or *obese* with various exceptions, such as: athletes, children, the elderly, and the infirm. Also, the growth of a child is documented against a BMI-measured growth chart. Obesity trends can then be calculated from the difference between the child's BMI and the BMI on the chart. In the United States, BMI is also used as a measure of underweight, owing to advocacy on behalf of those with eating disorders, such as anorexia nervosa and bulimia nervosa.

Legislation

In France, Israel, Italy and Spain, legislation has been introduced banning usage of fashion show models having a BMI below 18. In Israel, a BMI below 18.5 is banned. This is done in order to fight anorexia among models and people interested in fashion.

Limitations

The medical establishment and statistical community have both highlighted the limitations of BMI.

Mathematician Keith Devlin and the restaurant industry association Center for Consumer Freedom argue that the error in the BMI is significant and so pervasive that it is not generally useful in evaluation of health. University of Chicago political science professor Eric Oliver says BMI is a convenient but inaccurate measure of weight, forced onto the populace, and should be revised.

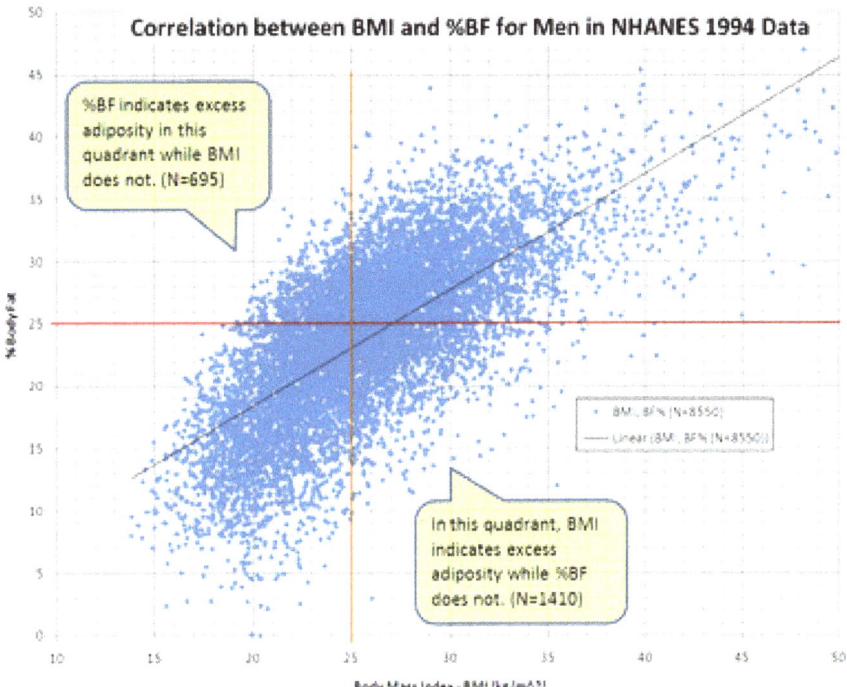

This graph shows the correlation between body mass index (BMI) and percent body fat (%BF) for 8550 men in NCHS' NHANES 1994 data. Data in the upper left and lower right quadrants suggest the limitations of BMI

Scaling

The exponent in the denominator of the formula for BMI is arbitrary. The BMI depends upon weight and the *square* of height. Since mass increases to the *3rd power* of linear dimensions, taller individuals with exactly the same body shape and relative composition have a larger BMI.

The mathematician Prof Nick Trefethen, who observed this said, "BMI divides the weight by too large a number for short people and too small a number for tall people. So short people are misled into thinking that they are thinner than they are, and tall people are misled into thinking they are fatter."

Sports medicine doctor Sultan M. Babar has shown that corpulence index is a better measure.

An analysis based on data gathered in the US suggested an exponent of 2.6 would yield the best fit for children aged 2 to 19 years old. For US adults, exponent estimates range from 1.92 to 1.96 for males and from 1.45 to 1.95 for females.

Ignores Variation in Physical Characteristics

The BMI adds roughly 10% for a large (or tall) frame and subtracts roughly 10% for a smaller frame (short stature). In other words, persons with small frames would be carrying more fat than optimal, but their BMI reflects that they are *normal*. Conversely, large framed (or tall) individuals may be quite healthy, with a fairly low body fat percentage, but be classified as *overweight* by BMI.

For example, a chart may say the ideal weight for a man 5 ft 10 in (178 cm) is 165 pounds (75 kg). But if that man has a slender build (small frame), he may be overweight at 165 pounds (75 kg) and should reduce by 10%, to roughly 150 pounds (68 kg). In the reverse, the man with a larger frame and more solid build can be quite healthy at 180 pounds (82 kg). If one teeters on the edge of small/medium or medium/large, common sense should be used in calculating one's ideal weight. However, falling into one's ideal weight range for height and build is still not as accurate in determining health risk factors as waist/height ratio and actual body fat percentage.

Accurate frame size calculators use several measurements (wrist circumference, elbow width, neck circumference and others) to determine what category an individual falls into for a given height. The BMI also fails to take into account loss of height through aging. In this situation, BMI will increase without any corresponding increase in weight.

Does not Differentiate between Muscle Mass and Fat Mass

Assumptions about the distribution between muscle mass and fat mass are inexact. BMI generally overestimates adiposity on those with more lean body mass (e.g., athletes) and underestimates excess adiposity on those with less lean body mass. A study in June 2008 by Romero-Corral et al. examined 13,601 subjects from the United States' third National Health and Nutrition Examination Survey (NHANES III) and found that BMI-defined obesity (BMI > 30) was present in 21% of men and 31% of women.

Using body fat percentages (BF%), however, BF-defined obesity was found in 50% of men and 62% of women. While BMI-defined obesity showed high specificity (95% for men and 99% for women), BMI showed poor sensitivity (36% for men and 49% for women). Despite this undercounting of obesity by BMI, BMI values in the intermediate BMI range of 20–30 were found to be associated with a wide range of body fat percentages. For men with a BMI of 25, about 20% have a body fat percentage below 20% and about 10% have body fat percentage above 30%.

BMI is particularly inaccurate for people who are very fit or athletic, as their high muscle mass can classify them in the *overweight* category by BMI, even though their body fat percentages frequently fall in the 10–15% category, which is below that of a more sedentary person of average build who has a *normal* BMI number. Body composition for athletes is often better calculated using measures of body fat, as determined by such techniques as skinfold measurements or underwater weighing and the limitations of manual measurement have also led to new, alternative methods to measure obesity, such as the body volume index.

Variation in Definitions of Categories

It is not clear where on the BMI scale the threshold for *overweight* and *obese* should be set. Because of this the standards have varied over the past few decades. Between 1980 and 2000 the U.S. Dietary Guidelines have defined overweight at a variety of levels ranging from a BMI of 24.9 to 27.1. In 1985 the National Institutes of Health (NIH) consensus conference recommended that overweight BMI be set at a BMI of 27.8 for men and 27.3 for women.

In 1998 a NIH report concluded that a BMI over 25 is overweight and a BMI over 30 is obese. In the 1990s the World Health Organization (WHO) decided that a BMI of 25 to 30 should be considered overweight and a BMI over 30 is obese, the standards the NIH set. This became the definitive guide for determining if someone is overweight.

The current WHO and NIH ranges of *normal* weights are proved to be associated with decreased risks of some diseases such as diabetes type II; however using the same range of BMI for men and women is considered arbitrary, and makes the definition of underweight quite unsuitable for men.

One study found that the vast majority of people labelled 'overweight' and 'obese' according to current definitions do not in fact face any meaningful increased risk for early death. In a quantitative analysis of a number of studies, involving more than 600,000 men and women, the lowest mortality rates were found for people with BMIs between 23 and 29; most of the 25–30 range considered 'overweight' was not associated with higher risk.

Variation in Relationship to Health

A study published by *Journal of the American Medical Association* (*JAMA*) in 2005 showed that *overweight* people had a death rate similar to *normal* weight people as defined by BMI, while *underweight* and *obese* people had a higher death rate.

A study published by *The Lancet* in 2009 involving 900,000 adults showed that *overweight* and *underweight* people both had a mortality rate higher than *normal* weight people as defined by BMI. The optimal BMI was found to be in the range of 22.5–25.

High BMI is associated with type 2 diabetes only in persons with high serum gamma-glutamyl transpeptidase.

In an analysis of 40 studies involving 250,000 people, patients with coronary artery disease with *normal* BMIs were at higher risk of death from cardiovascular disease than people whose BMIs put them in the *overweight* range (BMI 25–29.9).

One study found that BMI had a good general correlation with body fat percentage, and noted that obesity has overtaken smoking as the world's number one cause of death. But it also notes that in the study 50% of men and 62% of women were obese according to body fat defined obesity, while only 21% of men and 31% of women were obese according to BMI, meaning that BMI was found to underestimate the number of obese subjects.

A 2010 study that followed 11,000 subjects for up to eight years concluded that BMI is not a good measure for the risk of heart attack, stroke or death. A better measure was found to be the waist-to-height ratio. A 2011 study that followed 60,000 participants for up to 13 years found that waist–hip ratio was a better predictor of ischaemic heart disease mortality.

Alternatives

BMI Prime

BMI Prime, a modification of the BMI system, is the ratio of actual BMI to upper limit optimal BMI (currently defined at 25 kg/m²), i.e., the actual BMI expressed as a proportion of upper limit optimal. The ratio of actual body weight to body weight for upper limit optimal BMI (25 kg/m²) is equal to BMI Prime. BMI Prime is a dimensionless number independent of units. Individuals with BMI Prime less than 0.74 are underweight; those with between 0.74 and 1.00 have optimal weight; and those at 1.00 or greater are overweight. BMI Prime is useful clinically because it shows by what ratio (e.g. 1.36) or percentage (e.g. 136%, or 36% above) a person deviates from the maximum optimal BMI.

For instance, a person with BMI 34 kg/m² has a BMI Prime of 34/25 = 1.36, and is 36% over their upper mass limit. In South East Asian and South Chinese populations, BMI Prime should be calculated using an upper limit BMI of 23 in the denominator instead of 25. BMI Prime allows easy comparison between populations whose upper-limit optimal BMI values differ.

Waist Circumference

Waist circumference is a good indicator of visceral fat, which poses more health risks than fat elsewhere. According to the U.S. National Institutes of Health (NIH), waist circumference in excess of 102 centimetres (40 in) for men and 88 centimetres (35 in) for (non-pregnant) women, is considered to infer a high risk for type 2 diabetes, dyslipidemia, hypertension, and CVD. Waist circumference can be a better indicator of obesity-related disease risk than BMI. For example, this is the case in populations of Asian descent and older people. 94 centimetres (37 in) for men and 80 centimetres (31 in) for women has been stated to pose "higher risk", with the NIH figures "even higher".

Waist-to-hip circumference ratio has also been used, but has been found to be no better than waist circumference alone, but more complicated to measure.

A related indicator is waist circumference divided by height. The values indicating increased risk are: greater than 0.5 for people under 40 year of age, 0.5 to 0.6 for people aged 40–50, and greater than 0.6 for people over 50 years of age.

Surface-based Body Shape Index

The Surface-based Body Shape Index (SBSI) is far more rigorous and is based upon four key measurements: the body surface area, vertical trunk circumference, waist circumference and height. Data on 11,808 subjects from the National Health and Human Nutrition Examination Surveys (NHANES) 1999–2004, showed that SBSI outperformed BMI, waist circumference, and A Body Shape Index (ABSI), an alternative to BMI.

$$SBSI = \frac{(H^{7/4})(WC^{5/6})}{BSA\ VTC}$$

Modified Body Mass Index

Within some medical contexts, such as familial amyloid polyneuropathy, serum albumin is factored in to produce a modified body mass index (mBMI). The mBMI can be obtained by multiplying the BMI by serum albumin, in grams per litre.

References

- Bowling A (2005). "Mode of questionnaire administration can have serious effects on data quality". Journal of Public Health. 27 (3): 281–91. doi:10.1093/pubmed/fdi031. PMID 15870099

- Huettel, S. A.; Song, A. W.; McCarthy, G. (2009), Functional Magnetic Resonance Imaging (2 ed.), Massachusetts: Sinauer, ISBN 978-0-87893-286-3

- Bulte, D. (2006), BOLD Physiology (Lecture slides) (PDF), Center for FMRI of the Brain, University of Oxford, retrieved December 31, 2011

- Devlin, H. (2012), Introduction to fMRI: Clinical and commercial use, The Oxford Centre for Functional MRI of the Brain, University of Oxford, UK, retrieved January 1, 2012

- International Journal of Eating DisordersVolume 4 Issue 4, Pages 511 - 523 Published Online: 13 Feb 2006 Copyright © 2009 Wiley Periodicals, Inc., A Wiley Company Sense of ineffectiveness in women with eating disorders

- Raichle, M. E. (2000), Toga, A. W.; Mazziotta, J. C., eds., Brain mapping: the systems, London: Academic Press, ISBN 978-0-12-692545-6

- Cooper, Z; Fairburn, CG (1987). "The Eating Disorder Examination: A semistructured interview for the assessment of the specific psychopathology of eating disorders.". International Journal of Eating Disorders. 6: 1–8.

- Rombouts, S. A. R. B.; Barkhof, F.; Sheltens, P. (2007), Clinical applications of functional brain MRI, UK: Oxford University Press, ISBN 978-0-19-856629-8

- Functional MR Imaging (fMRI) - Brain, American College of Radiology & Radiological Society of North America, May 24, 2011, retrieved December 30, 2011

- Roy, C. S.; Sherrington, C. S. (1890), "On the regulation of the blood-supply of the brain", Journal of Physiology, 11 (1–2): 85–158, PMC 1514242, PMID 16991945

- Health risks from exposure to low levels of ionizing radiation : BEIR VII Phase. Washington, D.C.: National Academies Press. 2006. ISBN 978-0-309-09156-5

- "Response to the FDA's May 23, 2007, Nephrogenic Systemic Fibrosis Update1 — Radiology". Radiology.rsna.org. 2007-09-12. Retrieved 2010-08-02

- Leksell L; Leksell D; Schwebel J (1985). "Stereotaxis and nuclear magnetic resonance". Journal of Neurology, Neurosurgery & Psychiatry. 48 (1): 14–18. doi:10.1136/jnnp.48.1.14. PMC 1028176. PMID 3882889

- McRobbie, Donald W. (2007). MRI from picture to proton. Cambridge, UK ; New York: Cambridge University Press. ISBN 0-521-68384-X

- Thomas DG; Davis CH; Ingram S; Olney JS; Bydder GM; Young IR (1986). "Stereotaxic biopsy of the brain under MR imaging control". AJNR American Journal of Neuroradiology. 7 (1): 161–163. PMID 3082131

- Haacke, E Mark; Brown, Robert F; Thompson, Michael; Venkatesan, Ramesh (1999). Magnetic resonance imaging: Physical principles and sequence design. New York: J. Wiley & Sons. ISBN 0-471-35128-8

- "A SHORT HISTORY OF MAGNETIC RESONANCE IMAGING FROM A EUROPEAN POINT OF VIEW". emrf.org. Archived from the original on 2007-04-13. Retrieved 2016-08-08

4

Treatments for Eating Disorder

Cognitive behavioral therapy is the therapy given to patients with eating disorders in order to alter or reduce their negative thoughts. Other treatments given to patients emphasize the social, biological, psychological and emotional harm caused by the disorder. Eating disorder is best understood in confluence with the major topics listed in the following chapter.

Cognitive Behavioral Treatment of Eating Disorders

Cognitive behavioral therapy (CBT) is derived from both the cognitive and behavioral schools of psychology and focuses on the alteration of thoughts and actions with the goal of treating various disorders. The cognitive behavioral treatment of eating disorders emphasizes the minimization of negative thoughts about body image and the act of eating, and attempts to alter negative and harmful behaviors that are involved in and perpetuate eating disorders. It also encourages the ability to tolerate negative thoughts and feelings as well as the ability to think about food and body perception in a multi-dimensional way. The emphasis is not only placed on altering cognition, but also on tangible practices like making goals and being rewarded for meeting those goals. CBT is a "time-limited and focused approach" which means that it is important for the patients of this type of therapy to have particular issues that they want to address when they begin treatment. CBT has also proven to be one of the most effective treatments for eating disorders.

CBT-Enhanced

A common form of CBT that is used to treat eating disorders is called CBT-Enhanced (CBT-E) and was developed by Christopher G. Fairburn throughout the 1970s and 1980s. Originally intended for bulimia nervosa specifically, it was eventually extended to all eating disorders. Within Fairburn's enhanced CBT is CBT-Ef, designed to deal particularly with eating habits, and CBT-Eb for other issues that don't directly involve eating.

Bulimia Nervosa

A study conducted by the UK National Institute for Health and Clinical Excellence has found that CBT is the best treatment for bulimia nervosa. Enhanced CBT is delivered on an individual basis and usually in an outpatient situation and is meant to help with the psychopathology of the eating disorder rather than the diagnosis itself. Research demonstrates that antidepressants may be an effective alternative to CBT for treatment of eating disorders; however, CBT continues to prove more effective than antidepressants specifically for the treatment of bulimia nervosa. A small study on patients with bulimia combined CBT with text-messaging a therapist about the frequency of binge-purge behaviours and the strength of the patient's desires to binge and purge. The number of binge eating and purging episodes decreased significantly from base-line to post-treatment and followup.

Anorexia Nervosa

Less research has been conducted on the effectiveness of CBT for those with anorexia nervosa, but a recent study demonstrated that CBT was effective for 60% of the subjects tested – 60% of those for whom CBT was effective were improved upon receiving the treatment. In addition, the US National Guideline Clearinghouse reported that CBT can alleviate symptoms of depression and compulsivity that are associated with anorexia nervosa.

Binge-eating Disorder

The same type of CBT used for bulimia nervosa has demonstrated that it can be helpful in the treatment of binge-eating disorder. However, one of the problems with administering CBT to those suffering from this disorder is that it does not traditionally encourage weight loss. This can be problematic for binge-eaters who are overweight or obese. As a result of issues like these CBT has not yet been established as the most effective treatment for binge-eating disorder. A commonly used alternative is behavioral weight loss because it prioritizes physical health by maintaining a healthy weight.

Other Eating Disorders

Eating disorders not otherwise specified (NOS) have been given less attention than anorexia nervosa and bulimia nervosa which are given their own categories in the DSM-IV-TR. That said, a recent study has shown that CBT is just as effective for treating eating disorders NOS as it is for bulimia nervosa

Eating Recovery

Eating recovery refers to the full spectrum of care that acknowledges and treats the multiple etiologies of anorexia nervosa and bulimia, including the biological, psychological, social and emotional causes of the disorder, through a comprehensive, integrated treatment regimen. When successful, this regimen restores the individual to a healthy weight and arms him or her with the skills and resources needed to maintain a sustainable recovery. Although there are a variety of treatment options available to the eating disorders patient, the intensive and multi-faceted program followed in eating recovery is the appropriate option for individuals who require intensive support and are able to commit to treatment in an inpatient, residential or full-day hospital setting.

Eating recovery has been associated with increased likelihood of a sustained post-treatment recovery. This carefully orchestrated treatment curriculum incorporates the following tenets to help patients cultivate an understanding of disease-management skills and how to implement those lessons into their post-treatment lives.

Biological/Medical Treatment

Eating disorders are physically and emotionally destructive. Most individuals with an eating disorder require ongoing medical treatment throughout their recovery. According to the Eating Disorder Foundation, early diagnosis and intervention significantly enhance chances of recovery, while eating disorders that are not identified or treated in their early stages can become chronic, debilitating and life-threatening.

For most people with eating disorders, the medical complications associated with the disease can be successfully treated with a combination of ongoing medical care and monitoring, nutritional counseling and medication. The Eating Disorder Foundation recommends people with eating disorders seek a recovery option that involves clinicians from different health disciplines, such as nursing, nutrition and mental health, a treatment philosophy consistent with the tenets of eating recovery.

Medical issues associated with eating disorders. Extremely medically compromised patients who are at a very low weight will require a more intensive medical intervention. Anorexia patients with a very low body weight (BMI < 13) may need to be stabilized due to medical complications caused by starvation, including liver failure or heart problems. Bulimia patients may need to manage edema, hypokalemia or esophagitis.

Poor nutrition affects the brain's chemicals and functionality. As a result, extremely low weight patients will have difficulty responding to cognitive therapy without first gaining weight. Medically supervised weight restoration is necessary before psychotherapy or many pharmaceuticals can affect the patient's behavioral health.

Misdiagnosis of the medical complications of eating disorders is common due to the unique physiology of these patients. Eating disorders can slow a resting heart rate and lower a "normal" body temperature range. For this reason, patients should seek specialized care from a doctor experienced in treating eating disorders.

Mindfulness

During the process of eating recovery, patients integrate mindfulness into every area of their treatment. Mindfulness is a mental state, characterized by concentrated awareness of one's thoughts, actions or motivations. Being "present" in every element of treatment, including meals, therapy sessions, classes or medical treatment helps patients become more receptive to different points of view. It also helps them become less reactive to emotions, instead focusing only on activities occurring in the present moment.

Mindfulness training focused on eating, body image and body awareness can lead the way to health, and recovery by enabling individuals to consciously experience and observe their internal mental and bodily events as well as those external events that are perceived directly through the senses. In eating recovery, mindfulness helps patients calm their minds and understand their self-defeating emotions or mood-dependent behaviors and instead cultivate healthy coping skills.

Mindfulness facilitates two key techniques—*mentalizing* and *building self-awareness*.

Mentalization in eating recovery takes the concept of mindfulness one step further, often thought of as mindfulness of mind. Mentalization describes a person's ability to understand the mental state of him- or herself and others based on overt behavior. Mentalization is a core challenge among people with eating disorders, and its lack can result in severe emotional fluctuations, impulsivity, and vulnerability to interpersonal and social interactions, particularly in the midst of emotional interaction.

In eating recovery, patients work with their therapists to mentalize, or identify, their own emotions while understanding that others may hold differing points of view. The ability to understand emotions and see situations from more than one viewpoint reduces anxiety and minimizes the need to rely on an eating disorder as a coping mechanism.

Self-awareness refers to an individual's ability to become aware of their own subconscious thinking. Absence of self-awareness is frequently seen in eating disorder patients, causing them to react to situations, feelings and other stimuli emotionally rather than rationally.

By practicing mindful self-awareness, eating recovery learn to examine their thoughts, feelings, memories and bodily sensations from an objective point of view. Patients are encouraged to let go of self-centered thinking to achieve a state wherein individuals are able to observe their thoughts and understand their subconscious motivations—sexual, material, emotional, intellectual, and spiritual. This comprehension builds calmness and patience, minimizing the need to rely on an eating disorder as a coping mechanism.

Motivation

Motivation is the set of reasons that determines why and how individuals engage in particular behaviors. In eating recovery, the goal is to shift patients from emotion-motivated behavior to values-motivated behavior through self-directedness and the construction of values awareness. Patients learn to identify their own core values and direct themselves in behaviors that align with their value systems, while limiting behaviors that do not.

Driving self-directedness. Self-directedness is a dimension of a person's character which has to do with the ability of an individual to control, regulate, and adapt their behavior to the situation at hand in accordance with their own goals, purposes, and values. An individual's inability to curtail eating disorder behaviors stems from low self-directedness. Eating recovery focuses on helping patients engage in self-directed behavior by giving their actions meaning within a values context.

Building values awareness. Self-directedness is difficult, if not impossible, without awareness of core values. Values provide the context for actions and feelings. Without awareness of values, people are often swayed by their emotional responses which may or may not serve their long-range goals and purposes. Under the sway of emotions, eating disorder behavior may become impulsive, "automatic", and mindless.

In eating recovery, clinicians and therapists assist patients in identifying their core values. This approach allows patients to see the "big picture" and engage in behaviors that align with their core values while avoiding behaviors of a conflicting nature.

Mood Management

Chronic anxiety is a key trait of individuals with eating disorders, their lives consumed with coping with the emotions that result from anxiety. These emotion-driven moods often elicit negative coping behaviors and narrow the patient's awareness of coping options. These impulsive behaviors can drive mindless, rigid, stereotyped responses such those seen with eating disorders.

In eating recovery, cognitive behavioral therapy and dialectical behavioral therapy are employed to interrupt negative cycles of behavior and replace them with positive, purposeful coping mechanisms.

Cognitive behavioral therapy' or *CBT* is a psychotherapeutic approach utilized in eating recovery that aims to influence dysfunctional emotions, behaviors and cognitions through a goal-oriented, systematic procedure. Cognitive-behavioral therapy is used to treat the mental and emotional elements of an eating disorder, helping patients change their attitudes about food, eating, and body image, correct poor eating habits, and prevent relapse.

Dialectical behavioral therapy or *DBT* combines standard cognitive-behavioral techniques for emotion regulation and reality-testing with concepts of mindful awareness, distress tolerance, and acceptance in the treatment of eating disorders. Influenced by Buddhist meditative practice, DBT includes the following key elements: behaviorist theory, dialectics, cognitive therapy, and, DBT's central component, mindfulness.

Seeking Recovery

According to the Eating Disorder Foundation, eating disorders are serious and complex illnesses that require the attention of trained professionals. Although those with the disease may have the desire, it is almost impossible for "self treatment" to be effective; in fact, trying to go it alone will likely result in repeated failures. Early detection and intervention has been proven to increase the chance of full recovery. It is essential for the person with the illness to get a professional assessment first, from a practitioner trained in eating recovery.

Healthy Diet

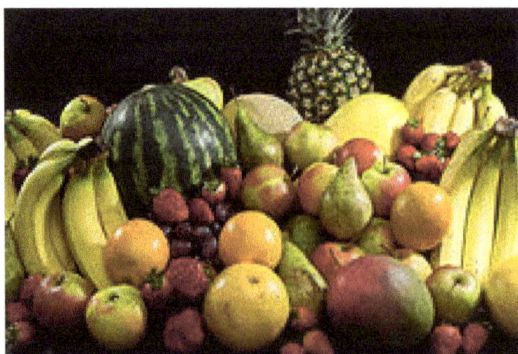

Common colorful culinary fruits. Apples, pears, strawberries, oranges, bananas grapes, canary melons, watermelon, cantaloupe, pineapple and mango.

A healthy diet is one that helps to maintain or improve overall health.

A healthy diet provides the body with essential nutrition: fluid, adequate essential amino acids from protein, essential fatty acids, vitamins, minerals, and adequate calories. The requirements for a healthy diet can be met from a variety of plant-based and animal-based foods. A healthy diet supports energy needs and provides for human nutrition without exposure to toxicity or excessive weight gain from consuming excessive amounts. Where lack of calories is not an issue, a properly balanced diet (in addition to exercise) is also thought to be important for lowering health risks, such as obesity, heart disease, type 2 diabetes, hypertension and cancer.

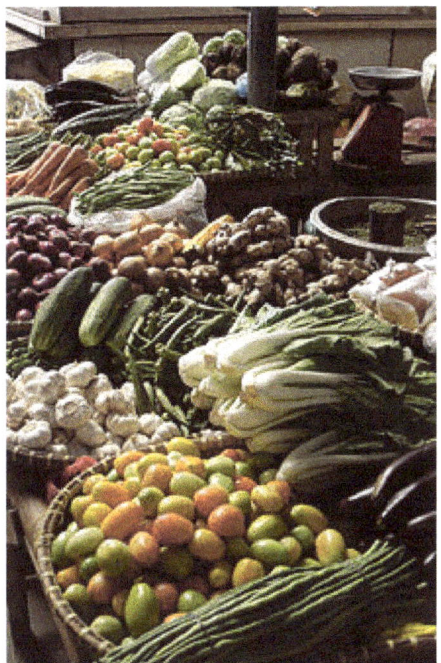

Leafy green, allium, and cruciferous vegetables are key components of a healthy diet

Various nutrition guides are published by medical and governmental institutions to educate the public on what they should be eating to promote health. Nutrition facts labels are also mandatory in some countries to allow consumers to choose between foods based on the components relevant to health.

The idea of dietary therapy (using dietary choices to maintain health and improve poor health) is quite old and thus has both modern scientific forms (medical nutrition therapy) and prescientific forms (such as dietary therapy in traditional Chinese medicine).

Mainstream Science

Healthy eating is simple, according to Marion Nestle, who expresses the mainstream view among scientists who study nutrition:

The basic principles of good diets are so simple that I can summarize them in just ten words: eat less, move more, eat lots of fruits and vegetables. For additional clarification, a five-word modifier helps: go easy on junk foods. Follow these precepts and you will go a long way toward preventing the major diseases of our overfed society—coronary heart disease, certain cancers, diabetes, stroke, osteoporosis, and a host of others.... These precepts constitute the bottom line of what seem to be the far more complicated dietary recommendations of many health organizations and national and international governments—the forty-one "key recommendations" of the 2005 Dietary Guidelines, for example. ... Although you may feel as though advice about nutrition is constantly changing, the basic ideas behind my four precepts have not changed in half a century. And they leave plenty of room for enjoying the pleasures of food.

David L. Katz, who reviewed the most prevalent popular diets in 2014, noted:

> The weight of evidence strongly supports a theme of healthful eating while allowing for variations on that theme. A diet of minimally processed foods close to nature, predominantly plants, is decisively associated with health promotion and disease prevention and is consistent with the salient components of seemingly distinct dietary approaches. Efforts to improve public health through diet are forestalled not for want of knowledge about the optimal feeding of Homo sapiens but for distractions associated with exaggerated claims, and our failure to convert what we reliably know into what we routinely do. Knowledge in this case is not, as of yet, power; would that it were so.

Recommendations

World Health Organization

The World Health Organization (WHO) makes the following 5 recommendations with respect to both populations and individuals:

- Eat roughly the same amount of calories that your body is using and maintain a healthy weight.

- Limit intake of fats, and prefer unsaturated fats to saturated fats and trans fats.

- Increase consumption of plant foods, particularly fruits, vegetables, legumes, whole grains and nuts.

- Limit the intake of sugar. A 2003 report recommends less than 10% of calorie intake from simple sugars.

- Limit salt / sodium consumption from all sources and ensure that salt is iodized.

Other recommendations include:

- Essential micronutrients such as vitamins and certain minerals.

- Avoiding directly poisonous (e.g. heavy metals) and carcinogenic (e.g. benzene) substances.

- Avoiding foods contaminated by human pathogens (e.g. *E. coli*, tapeworm eggs).

WHO recommends an intake of less than 5 grams of salt per day for the prevention of cardiovascular disease.

United States Department of Agriculture

The Dietary Guidelines for Americans by the United States Department of Agriculture (USDA) recommends three healthy patterns of diet, summarized in table below, for a 2000 kcal diet.

It emphasizes both health and environmental sustainability and a flexible approach: the committee that drafted it wrote: "The major findings regarding sustainable diets were that a diet higher in plant-based foods, such as vegetables, fruits, whole grains, legumes, nuts, and seeds, and lower in calories and animal-based foods is more health promoting and is associated with less environmental impact than is the current U.S. diet. This pattern of eating can be achieved through a variety of dietary patterns, including the "Healthy U.S.-style Pattern," the "Healthy Mediterranean-style Pattern," and the "Healthy Vegetarian Pattern". Food group amounts per day, unless noted per week.

Food group/subgroup (units)	Healthy US patterns	Healthy Vegetarian patterns	Healthy Med-style patterns
Fruits (cup eq)	2	2	2.5
Vegetables (cup eq)	2.5	2.5	2.5
Dark green	1.5/wk	1.5/wk	1.5/wk
Red/orange	5.5/wk	5.5/wk	5.5/wk
Starchy	5/wk	5/wk	5/wk
Legumes	1.5/wk	3/wk	1.5/wk
Others	4/wk	4/wk	4/wk
Grains (oz eq)	6	6.5	6
Whole	3	3.5	3
Refined	3	3	3
Dairy (cup eq)	3	3	2
Protein Foods (oz eq)	5.5	3.5	6.5
Meat (red and processed)	12.5/wk	--	12.5/wk
Poultry	10.5/wk	--	10.5/wk
Seafood	8/wk	--	15/wk
Eggs	3/wk	3/wk	3/wk
Nuts/seeds	4/wk	7/wk	4/wk
Processed Soy (including tofu)	0.5/wk	8/wk	0.5/wk
Oils (grams)	27	27	27
Solid fats limit (grams)	18	21	17
Added sugars limit (grams)	30	36	29

American Heart Association / World Cancer Research Fund / American Institute for Cancer Research

The American Heart Association, World Cancer Research Fund, and American Institute for Cancer Research recommend a diet that consists mostly of unprocessed plant foods, with emphasis a wide range of whole grains, legumes, and non-starchy vegetables and fruits. This healthy diet is full of a wide range of various non-starchy vegetables and fruits, that provide different colors including red, green, yellow, white, purple, and orange. They note that tomato cooked with oil, allium vegetables like garlic, and cruciferous vegetables like cauliflower, provide some protection against cancer. This healthy diet is low in energy density, which may protect against weight gain and associated diseases. Finally, limiting consumption of sugary drinks, limiting energy rich foods, including "fast foods" and red meat, and avoiding processed meats improves health and longevity. Overall, researchers and medical policy conclude that this healthy diet can reduce the risk of chronic disease and cancer.

In children, consuming less than 25 grams of added sugar (100 calories) is recommended per day. Other recommendations include no extra sugars in those under 2 years old and less than one soft drink per week. As of 2017, decreasing total fat is no longer recommended, but instead, the recommendation to lower risk of cardiovascular disease is to increase consumption of monounsaturated fats and polyunsaturated fats, while decreasing consumption of saturated fats.

Harvard School of Public Health

The Nutrition Source of Harvard School of Public Health makes the following 10 recommendations for a healthy diet:

- Choose good carbohydrates: whole grains (the less processed the better), vegetables, fruits and beans. Avoid white bread, white rice, and the like as well as pastries, sugared sodas, and other highly processed food.

- Pay attention to the protein package: good choices include fish, poultry, nuts, and beans. Try to avoid red meat.

- Choose foods containing healthy fats. Plant oils, nuts, and fish are the best choices. Limit consumption of saturated fats, and avoid foods with trans fat.

- Choose a fiber-filled diet which includes whole grains, vegetables, and fruits.

- Eat more vegetables and fruits—the more colorful and varied, the better.

- Calcium is important, but milk is not its best or only source. Good sources of calcium are collards, bok choy, fortified soy milk, baked beans, and supplements which contain calcium and vitamin D.

- Water is the best source of liquid. Avoid sugary drinks, and limit intake of juices and milk. Coffee, tea, artificially-sweetened drinks, 100-percent fruit juices, low-fat milk and alcohol can fit into a healthy diet but are best consumed in moderation. Sports drinks are recommended only for people who exercise more than an hour at a stretch to replace substances lost in sweat.

- Limit salt intake. Choose more fresh foods, instead of processed ones.

- Moderate alcohol drinking has health benefits, but is not recommended for everyone.

- Daily multivitamin and extra vitamin D intake has potential health benefits.

Other than nutrition, the guide recommends frequent physical exercise and maintaining a healthy body weight.

For Specific Conditions

In addition to dietary recommendations for the general population, there are many specific diets that have primarily been developed to promote better health in specific population groups, such as people with high blood pressure (as in low sodium diets or the more specific DASH diet), or people who are overweight or obese (in weight control diets). However, some of them may have more or less evidence for beneficial effects in normal people as well.

Hypertension

A low sodium diet is beneficial for people with high blood pressure. A Cochrane review published in 2008 concluded that a long term (more than 4 weeks) low sodium diet has a useful effect to reduce blood pressure, both in people with hypertension and in people with normal blood pressure.

The DASH diet (Dietary Approaches to Stop Hypertension) is a diet promoted by the National Heart, Lung, and Blood Institute (part of the NIH, a United States government organization) to control hypertension. A major feature of the plan is limiting intake of sodium, and it also generally encourages the consumption of nuts, whole grains, fish, poultry, fruits and vegetables while lowering the consumption of red meats, sweets, and sugar. It is also "rich in potassium, magnesium, and calcium, as well as protein".

The Mediterranean diet has also been shown to improve cardiovascular outcomes.

Obesity

Weight control diets aim to maintain a controlled weight. In most cases dieting is used in combination with physical exercise to lose weight in those who are overweight or obese.

Diets to promote weight loss are divided into four categories: low-fat, low-carbohydrate, low-calorie, and very low calorie. A meta-analysis of six randomized controlled trials found no difference between the main diet types (low calorie, low carbohydrate, and low fat), with a 2–4 kilogram weight loss in all studies. At two years, all calorie-reduced diet types cause equal weight loss irrespective of the macronutrients emphasized.

Reduced Disease Risk

There may be a relationship between lifestyle including food consumption and potentially lowering the risk of cancer or other chronic diseases. A diet high in fruits and vegetables appears to decrease the risk of cardiovascular disease and death but not cancer.

A healthy diet may consist mostly of whole plant foods, with limited consumption of energy dense foods, red meat, alcoholic drinks and salt while reducing consumption of sugary drinks, and processed meat. A healthy diet may contain non-starchy vegetables and fruits, including those with red, green, yellow, white, purple or orange pigments. Tomato cooked with oil, allium vegetables like garlic, and cruciferous vegetables like cauliflower "probably" contain compounds which are under research for their possible anti-cancer activity.

A healthy diet is low in energy density, lowering caloric content, thereby possibly inhibiting weight gain and lowering risk against chronic diseases. Chronic Western diseases are associated with pathologically increased IGF-1 levels. Findings in molecular biology and epidemiologic data suggest that milk consumption is a promoter of chronic diseases of Western nations, including atherosclerosis, carcinogenesis and neurodegenerative diseases.

Unhealthy Diets

The Western pattern diet which is typically eaten by Americans and increasingly adapted by people in the developing world as they leave poverty is unhealthy: it is "rich in red meat, dairy products, processed and artificially sweetened foods, and salt, with minimal intake of fruits, vegetables, fish, legumes, and whole grains."

An unhealthy diet is a major risk factor for a number of chronic diseases including: high blood pressure, diabetes, abnormal blood lipids, overweight/obesity, cardiovascular diseases, and cancer.

The WHO estimates that 2.7 million deaths are attributable to a diet low in fruits and vegetables every year. Globally it is estimated to cause about 19% of gastrointestinal cancer, 31% of ischaemic heart disease, and 11% of strokes, thus making it one of the leading preventable causes of death worldwide.

Popular Diets

Popular diets, often referred to as fad diets, make promises of weight loss or other health advantages such as longer life without backing by solid science, and in many cases are characterized by highly restrictive or unusual food choices. Celebrity endorsements (including celebrity doctors) are frequently associated with popular diets, and the individuals who develop and promote these programs often profit handsomely.

Public Health

Fears of high cholesterol were frequently voiced up until the mid-1990s. However, more recent research has shown that the distinction between high- and low-density lipoprotein ('good' and 'bad' cholesterol, respectively) must be addressed when speaking of the potential ill effects of cholesterol. Different types of dietary fat have different effects on blood levels of cholesterol. For example, polyunsaturated fats tend to decrease both types of cholesterol; monounsaturated fats tend to lower LDL and raise HDL; saturated fats tend to either raise HDL, or raise both HDL and LDL; and trans fat tend to raise LDL and lower HDL.

While dietary cholesterol is only found in animal products such as meat, eggs, and dairy, studies have not found a link between eating cholesterol and blood levels of cholesterol.

Vending machines in particular have come under fire as being avenues of entry into schools for junk food promoters. However, there is little in the way of regulation and it is difficult for most people to properly analyze the real merits of a company referring to itself as "healthy." Recently, the Committee of Advertising Practice in the United Kingdom launched a proposal to limit media advertising for food and soft drink products high in fat, salt or sugar. The British Heart Foundation released its own government-funded advertisements, labeled "Food4Thought", which were targeted at children and adults to discourage unhealthy habits of consuming junk food.

Cultural and Psychological Factors

From a psychological and cultural perspective, a healthier diet may be difficult to achieve for people with poor eating habits. This may be due to tastes acquired in childhood and preferences for sugary, salty and/or fatty foods.

Dieting

Dieting is the practice of eating food in a regulated and supervised fashion to decrease, maintain, or increase body weight. In other words, it is conscious control or restriction of the diet. A restricted diet is often used by those who are overweight or obese, sometimes in combination with physical exercise, to reduce body weight. Some people follow a diet to gain weight (usually in the form of muscle). Diets can also be used to maintain a stable body weight and improve health. In particular, diets can be designed to prevent or treat diabetes.

Diets to promote weight loss can be categorized as: low-fat, low-carbohydrate, low-calorie, very low calorie and more recently flexible dieting. A meta-analysis of six randomized controlled trials found no difference between low-calorie, low-carbohydrate, and low-fat diets, with a 2–4 kilogram weight loss over 12–18 months in all studies. At two years, all calorie-reduced diet types cause equal weight loss irrespective of the macronutrients emphasized. In general, the most effective diet is any which reduces calorie consumption.

A study published in *American Psychologist* found that short-term dieting involving "severe restriction of calorie intake" does not lead to "sustained improvements in weight and health for the majority of individuals". Other studies have found that the average individual maintains some weight loss after dieting. Weight loss by dieting, while of benefit to those classified as unhealthy, may slightly increase the mortality rate for individuals who are otherwise healthy.

The first popular diet was "Banting", named after William Banting. In his 1863 pamphlet, *Letter on Corpulence, Addressed to the Public*, he outlined the details of a particular low-carbohydrate, low-calorie diet that had led to his own dramatic weight loss.

History

One of the first dietitians was the English doctor George Cheyne. He himself was tremendously overweight and would constantly eat large quantities of rich food and drink. He began a meatless diet, taking only milk and vegetables, and soon regained his health. He began publicly recommending his diet for everyone suffering from obesity. In 1724, he wrote *An Essay of Health and Long Life*, in which he advises exercise and fresh air and avoiding luxury foods.

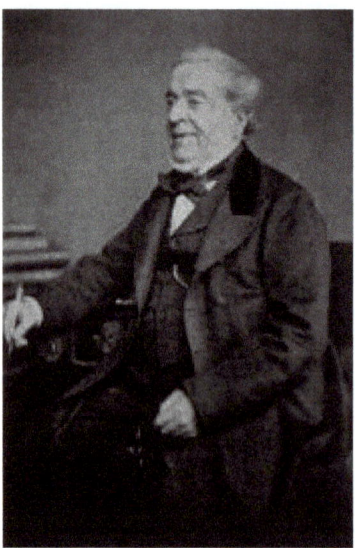

William Banting, popularized one of the first weight loss diets in the 19th century.

The Scottish military surgeon, John Rollo, published *Notes of a Diabetic Case* in 1797. It described the benefits of a meat diet for those suffering from diabetes, basing this recommendation on Matthew Dobson's discovery of glycosuria in diabetes mellitus. By means of Dobson's testing procedure (for glucose in the urine) Rollo worked out a diet that had success for what is now called type 2 diabetes.

The first popular diet was "Banting", named after the English undertaker William Banting. In 1863, he wrote a booklet called *Letter on Corpulence, Addressed to the Public,* which contained the particular plan for the diet he had successfully followed. His own diet was four meals per day, consisting of meat, greens, fruits, and dry wine. The emphasis was on avoiding sugar, sweet foods, starch, beer, milk and butter. Banting's pamphlet was popular for years to come, and would be used as a model for modern diets. The pamphlet's popularity was such that the question "Do you bant?" referred to his method, and eventually to dieting in general. His booklet remains in print as of 2007.

The first weight-loss book to promote calorie counting, and the first weight-loss book to become a bestseller, was the 1918 *Diet and Health: With Key to the Calories* by American physician and columnist Lulu Hunt Peters.

The Atkins Diet was suggested by the American nutritionist Robert Atkins in 1958, in a research paper titled "Weight Reduction". Atkins used the study to resolve his own overweight condition and went on to popularize the method in a series of books, starting with *Dr. Atkins' Diet Revolution* in 1972. In his second book, *Dr. Atkins' New Diet Revolution* (1992), he modified parts of the diet but did not alter the original concepts.

Types

Low-fat

Low-fat diets involve the reduction of the percentage of fat in one's diet. Calorie consumption is reduced because less fat is consumed. Diets of this type include NCEP Step I and II. A meta-analysis of 16 trials of 2–12 months' duration found that low-fat diets (without intentional restriction of caloric intake) resulted in average weight loss of 3.2 kg (7.1 lb) over habitual eating.

Low-carbohydrate

Low-carbohydrate diets such as Atkins and Protein Power are relatively high in protein and fats. Low-carbohydrate diets are sometimes *ketogenic* (i.e., they restrict carbohydrate intake sufficiently to cause ketosis).

Low-calorie

Low-calorie diets usually produce an energy deficit of 500–1,000 calories per day, which can result in a 0.5 to 1 kilogram (1.1 to 2.2 pounds) weight loss per week. Some of the most commonly used low-calorie diets include DASH diet and Weight Watchers. The National Institutes of Health reviewed 34 randomized controlled trials to determine the effectiveness of low-calorie diets. They found that these diets lowered total body mass by 8% in the short term, over 3–12 months. Women doing low-calorie diets should have at least 1,200 calories per day. Men should have at least 1,800 calories per day.

Very low-calorie

Very low calorie diets provide 200–800 calories per day, maintaining protein intake but limiting calories from both fat and carbohydrates. They subject the body to starvation and produce an average loss of 1.5–2.5 kg (3.3–5.5 lb) per week. "2-4-6-8", a popular diet of this variety, follows a four-day cycle in which only 200 calories are consumed the first day, 400 the second day, 600 the third day, 800 the fourth day, and then totally fasting, after which the cycle repeats. These diets are not recommended for general use as they are associated with adverse side effects such as loss of lean muscle mass, increased risks of gout, and electrolyte imbalances. People attempting these diets must be monitored closely by a physician to prevent complications.

Detox

Detox diets claim to eliminate "toxins" from the human body rather than claiming to cause weight loss. Many of these use herbs or celery and other juicy low-calorie vegetables.

Religious

Religious prescription may be a factor in motivating people to adopt a specific restrictive diet. For example, the Biblical Book of Daniel (1:2-20, and 10:2-3) refers to a 10- or 21-day avoidance of foods (Daniel Fast) declared unclean by God in the laws of Moses. In modern versions of the Daniel Fast, food choices may be limited to whole grains, fruits, vegetables, pulses, nuts, seeds and oil. The Daniel Fast resembles the vegan diet in that it excludes foods of animal origin. The passages strongly suggest that the Daniel Fast will promote good health and mental performance.

Fasting is practiced in various religions. Examples include Lent in Christianity; Yom Kippur, Tisha B'av, Fast of Esther, Tzom Gedalia, the Seventeenth of Tamuz, and the Tenth of Tevet in Judaism. Muslims refrain from eating during the hours of daytime for one entire month, Ramadan, every year.

Details of fasting practices differ. Eastern Orthodox Christians fast during specified fasting seasons of the year, which include not only the better-known Great Lent, but also fasts on every Wednesday and Friday (except on special holidays), together with extended fasting periods before Christmas (the Nativity Fast), after Easter (the Apostles Fast) and in early August (the Dormition Fast). Members of The Church of Jesus Christ of Latter-day Saints (Mormons) generally fast for 24 hours on the first Sunday of each month. Like Muslims, they refrain from all drinking and eating unless they are children or are physically unable to fast. Fasting is also a feature of ascetic traditions in religions such as Hinduism and Buddhism. Mahayana traditions that follow the Brahma's Net Sutra may recommend that the laity fast "during the six days of fasting each month and the three months of fasting each year" [Brahma's Net Sutra, minor precept 30]. Members of the Baha'i Faith observe a Nineteen Day Fast from sunrise to sunset during March each year.

Nutrition

Weight loss diets that manipulate the proportion of macronutrients (low-fat, low-carbohydrate, etc.) have been shown to be more effective than diets that maintain a typical mix of foods with smaller portions and perhaps some substitutions (e.g. low-fat milk, or less salad dressing). Extreme diets may, in some cases, lead to malnutrition.

Nutritionists also agree on the importance of avoiding fats, especially saturated fats, to reduce weight and to be healthier. They also agree on the importance of reducing salt intake because foods including snacks, biscuits, and bread already contain ocean-salt, contributing to an excess of salt daily intake.

MyPyramid Food Guidance System is the result of extensive research performed by the United States Department of Agriculture to revise the original Food Guide Pyramid. It offers a wide array of personalized options to help individuals make healthy food choices. It also provides advice on physical activity.

One of the most important things to take into consideration when either trying to lose or put on weight is output versus input. It is important to know the amount of energy your body is using every day, so that your intake fits the needs of one's personal weight goal. Someone wanting to lose weight would want a smaller energy intake than what they put out. There is increasing research-based evidence that low-fat vegetarian diets consistently lead to healthy weight loss and management, a decrease in diabetic symptoms as well as improved cardiac health.

How the Body Eliminates Fat

When the body is expending more energy than it is consuming (e.g. when exercising), the body's cells rely on internally stored energy sources, such as complex carbohydrates and fats, for energy. The first source to which the body turns is glycogen (by glycogenolysis). Glycogen is a complex carbohydrate, 65% of which is stored in skeletal muscles and the remainder in the liver (totaling about 2,000 kcal in the whole body). It is created from the excess of ingested macronutrients, mainly carbohydrates. When glycogen is nearly depleted, the body begins lipolysis, the mobilization and catabolism of fat stores for energy. In this process, fats, obtained from adipose tissue, or fat cells, are broken down into glycerol and fatty acids, which can be used to generate energy. The primary by-products of metabolism are carbon dioxide and water; carbon dioxide is expelled through the respiratory system.

Weight Loss Groups

Some weight loss groups aim to make money, others work as charities. The former include Weight Watchers and Peertrainer. The latter include Overeaters Anonymous and groups run by local organizations.

These organizations' customs and practices differ widely. Some groups are modelled on twelve-step programs, while others are quite informal. Some groups advocate certain prepared foods or special menus, while others train dieters to make healthy choices from restaurant menus and while grocery-shopping and cooking.

Food Diary

A 2008 study published in the American Journal of Preventive Medicine showed that dieters who kept a daily food diary (or diet journal), lost twice as much weight as those who did not keep a food log, suggesting that if you record your eating, you wouldn't eat as many calories.

Possible Weight Loss Effects of Drinking Water Prior to Meals

A 2009 review found that existing limited evidence suggested that encouraging water consumption and substituting energy-free beverages for energy-containing beverages (i.e., reducing caloric intake) may facilitate weight management. A 2009 article found that drinking 500 ml of water prior to meals for a 12-week period resulted in increased long-term weight reduction.

Fasting

Lengthy fasting can be dangerous due to the risk of malnutrition and should be carried out only under medical supervision. During prolonged fasting or very low calorie diets the reduction of blood glucose, the preferred energy source of the brain, causes the body to deplete its glycogen stores. Once glycogen is depleted the body begins to fuel the brain using ketones, while also metabolizing body protein (including but not limited to skeletal muscle) to be used to synthesize sugars for use as energy by the rest of the body. Most experts believe that a prolonged fast can lead to muscle wasting, although some dispute this. The use of short-term fasting, or various forms of intermittent fasting have been used as a form of dieting to circumvent this issue.

Side Effects

While there are studies that show the health and medical benefits of weight loss, a study in 2005 of around 3000 Finns over an 18-year period showed that weight loss from dieting can result in increased mortality, while those who maintained their weight fared the best. Similar conclusion is drawn by other studies, and although other studies suggest that intentional weight loss has a small benefit for individuals classified as unhealthy, it is associated with slightly increased mortality for healthy individuals and the slightly overweight but not obese. This may reflect the loss of subcutaneous fat and beneficial mass from organs and muscle in addition to visceral fat when there is a sudden and dramatic weight loss.

Low Carbohydrate Versus Low Fat

Many studies have focused on diets that reduce calories via a low-carbohydrate (Atkins diet, Scarsdale diet, Zone diet) diet versus a low-fat diet (LEARN diet, Ornish diet). The Nurses' Health Study, an observational cohort study, found that low carbohydrate diets based on vegetable sources of fat and protein are associated with less coronary heart disease. The same study also found no correlation (with multivariate adjustment) between animal fat intake and coronary heart disease (table 4). A long term study that monitored 43,396 Swedish women however suggests that a low carbohydrate-high protein diet, used on a regular basis and without consideration of the nature of carbohydrates or the source of proteins, is associated with increased risk of cardiovascular disease.

A meta-analysis of randomized controlled trials by the international Cochrane Collaboration in 2002 concluded that fat-restricted diets are no better than calorie-restricted diets in achieving long term weight loss in overweight or obese people. A more recent meta-analysis that included randomized controlled trials published after the Cochrane review found that low-carbohydrate, non-energy-restricted diets appear to be at least as effective as low-fat, energy-restricted diets in inducing weight loss for up to 1 year. These results can be understood because weight loss is mainly governed by daily caloric deficit and not by the particular foods eaten. However, when low-carbohydrate diets to induce weight loss are considered, potential favorable changes in triglyceride and high-density lipoprotein cholesterol values should be weighed against potential unfavorable changes in low-density lipoprotein cholesterol values."

The Women's Health Initiative Randomized Controlled Dietary Modification Trial found that a diet of total fat to 20% of energy and increasing consumption of vegetables and fruit to at least 5 servings daily and grains to at least 6 servings daily resulted in:

- no reduction in cardiovascular disease

- no statistically significant reduction in invasive breast cancer

- no reductions in colorectal cancer

Additional randomized controlled trials found that:

- A comparison of Atkins, Zone diet, Ornish diet, and LEARN diet in *premenopausal women* found the greatest benefit from the Atkins diet.

- The choice of diet for a specific person may be influenced by measuring the individual's insulin secretion:

  In young adults "Reducing glycemic [carbohydrate] load may be especially important to achieve weight loss among individuals with high insulin secretion." This is consistent with prior studies of diabetic patients in which low carbohydrate diets were more beneficial.

The American Diabetes Association recommended a low carbohydrate diet to reduce weight for those with or at risk of Type 2 diabetes in its January 2008 Clinical Practice Recommendations.

Low Glycemic Index

"The glycemic index (GI) factor is a ranking of foods based on their overall effect on blood sugar levels. The diet based around this research is called the Low GI diet. Low glycemic index foods, such as lentils, provide a slower, more consistent source of glucose to the bloodstream, thereby stimulating less insulin release than high glycemic index foods, such as white bread."

The glycemic load is "the mathematical product of the glycemic index and the carbohydrate amount".

In a randomized controlled trial that compared four diets that varied in carbohydrate amount and glycemic index found complicated results:

- Diet 1 and 2 were high carbohydrate (55% of total energy intake)

  o Diet 1 was high-glycemic index

  o Diet 2 was low-glycemic index

- Diet 3 and 4 were high protein (25% of total energy intake)

  o Diet 3 was high-glycemic index

  o Diet 4 was low-glycemic index

Diets 2 and 3 lost the most weight and fat mass; however, low density lipoprotein fell in Diet 2 and rose in Diet 3. Thus the authors concluded that the high-carbohydrate, low-glycemic index diet was the most favorable.

A meta-analysis by the Cochrane Collaboration concluded that low glycemic index or low glycemic load diets led to more weight loss and better lipid profiles. *However*, the Cochrane Collaboration grouped low glycemic index and low glycemic load diets together and did not try to separate the effects of the load versus the index.

Bland Diet

A bland diet is a diet consisting of foods that are generally soft, low in dietary fiber, cooked rather than raw, and not spicy. Fried and fatty foods, strong cheeses, whole grains (rich in fiber), and the medications aspirin and ibuprofen are also avoided while on this diet. Such a diet is called bland because it is soothing to the digestive tract (it minimizes irritation of tissues). It can also be bland in the sense of "lacking flavor", but it does not always have to be so; nonirritating food can be appetizing food, depending on preparation and individual preferences.

Uses

Bland diets are often recommended following stomach or intestinal surgery, or for people with ulcers, heartburn, nausea, vomiting, and gas. A bland diet allows the digestive tract to heal before introducing more difficult to digest foods.

Many milk and dairy products are permissible, even recommended, on a bland diet, but there are a few exceptions. Chocolate-flavored dairy products are discouraged, as well as any strongly spiced cheeses or high fat dairy products such as heavy cream or half-and-half. Mild dairy foods tend to soothe irritated linings, but excessive fats, cocoa and spices can have the opposite effect.

Most canned fruits and vegetables are fine, with the exception of tomatoes. Tomato-based sauces on pasta are avoided. Bananas are good, however, higher fiber and acidic fruits should be avoided. Baked potatoes and sweet potatoes are very easily digested, but it is important to avoid high fat toppings like butter. Vinegar based foods such as pickles are to be avoided as are sour fermented foods like sauerkraut.

Perhaps, the most difficult adjustment for some to a bland diet may involve meats and proteins. In a strict bland food diet, softer protein sources such as smooth peanut butter, eggs and tofu are encouraged over any type of fibrous or seasoned meat. Certain meats such as poultry or fish are permitted, as long as they are not heavily fried, breaded or processed like sandwich meats. Steamed poultry breast served with a salt substitute would be a typical protein serving while on a bland diet.

A bland diet is designed primarily to help patients recover from gastrointestinal conditions or other medical circumstances in which improved digestion would be essential. It is not especially effective as a long-term weight loss diet, although portion sizes are strictly controlled. Many people find a bland diet to be very difficult to maintain, although some find the use of acceptable spice alternatives does make it easier. Most patients slowly return to a more normal diet once their medical issues have been resolved.

Healthy Eating Pyramid

THE HEALTHY EATING PYRAMID

Department of Nutrition, Harvard School of Public Health

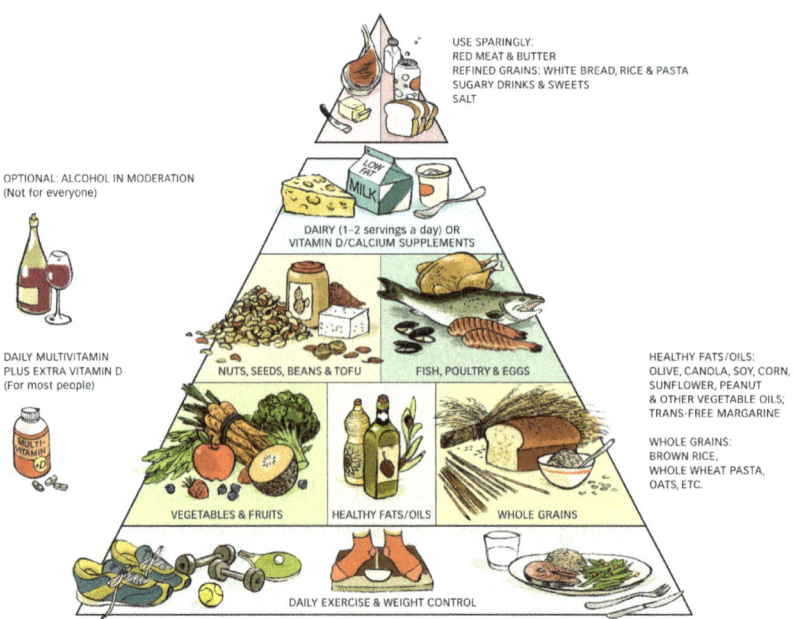

The Healthy Eating Pyramid (alternately, Healthy Eating Plate) is a nutrition guide developed by the Harvard School of Public Health, suggesting quantities of each food category that a human should eat each day. The healthy eating pyramid is intended to provide a sound eating guide than the widespread food guide pyramid created by the USDA.

The new pyramid aims to include more recent research in dietary health not present in the USDA's 1992 guide. The original USDA pyramid has been criticized for not differentiating between refined grains and whole grains, between saturated fats and unsaturated fats, and for not placing enough emphasis on exercise and weight control.

Food Groups

In general terms, the healthy eating pyramid recommends the following intake of different food groups each day, although exact amounts of calorie intake depends on sex, age, and lifestyle:

- At most meals, whole grain foods including oatmeal, whole-wheat bread, and brown rice; 1 piece or 4 ounces (110 g).

- Plant oils, including olive oil, canola oil, soybean oil, corn oil, and sunflower seed oil; 2 ounces (60 g) per day

- Vegetables, in abundance 3 or more each day; each serving = 6 ounces (170 g).

- 2–3 servings of fruits; each serving = 1 piece of fruit or 4 ounces (110 g).

- 1–3 servings of nuts, or legumes; each serving = 2 ounces (60 g).

- 1–2 servings of dairy or calcium supplement; each serving = 8 ounces (230 g) non fat or 4 ounces (110 g) of whole.

- 1–2 servings of poultry, fish, or eggs; each serving = 4 ounces (110 g) or 1 egg.

- Sparing use of white rice, white bread, potatoes, pasta and sweets;

- Sparing use of red meat and butter.

Intuitive Eating

Intuitive eating is a nutrition philosophy based on the premise that becoming more attuned to the body's natural hunger signals is a more effective way to attain a healthy weight, rather than keeping track of the amounts of energy and fats in foods. It's a process that is intended to create a healthy relationship with food, mind and body, making it a popular treatment for disordered eating and eating disorders.

Intuitive eating goes by many names, including non-dieting or the non-diet approach, normal eating, wisdom eating, and conscious eating. Some strategies and goals for building intuitive eating skills are discovering how to listen and reconnect with your body's hunger and fullness cues, learn to trust yourself to make decisions around what or how much to eat, take back your power around food, reconnect to your body's innate wisdom to determine the right amount of food for you, develop self-trust around eating challenging or "forbidden" foods, practice being more mindful at meal times in a safe and supportive environment. This approach to eating fights against weight stigma in terms of negative judgement, bias, assumptions, attitudes, and treatment based on a person's size. This stigma inevitably makes people feel worse about themselves and leads to even worse health outcomes for that individual.

"Weight neutrality" is a key component to intuitive eating because it is the process of making absolutely no assumptions about a person's health or habits based on physical appearance (weight in particular). It deems every individual deserving of health enhancing interventions regardless of whether it produces a change in weight. This leads to an intuitive eating approach that is critical to helping without harming.

"Health selfishness" is a term that can help explain the principles of intuitive eating because it includes the process of becoming clear on what food you need, owning what food you need whenever possible, and not apologizing for it. In short, it's about becoming attuned to your own sense of what is right for you. Furthermore, the process of intuitive eating more often than not leads to body positivity and an overwhelming acceptance of one's body, shape, and weight. Body positivity does not worry whether improved self-care results in weight loss because every body is different. Sometimes improved self-care leads to body changes and sometimes it does not. Body positivity is being your own unique self, not making changes to make yourself look like every other idealized image. Through intuitive eating, health selfishness, and body positivity, one can reach one's unique and full health potential without surrendering to society's idea of beauty or hurting themselves physically and emotionally.

History

Intuitive eating is not a recent idea. Aristotle is thought to have had some sort of intuitive eating and exercising philosophy by stating, "For both excessive and insufficient exercise destroy one's strength, and both eating and drinking too much or too little destroy health, whereas the right quantity produces, increases or preserves it." Horace Fletcher, a nineteenth-century health food enthusiast, advised eating only when hungry. Early twentieth-century self-help writer Wallace D. Wattles also encouraged eating only when one is hungry, and stop eating when hunger begins to abate.

Exactly when the intuitive eating movement began is uncertain, but one of the early pioneers was Susie Orbach, whose book *Fat is a Feminist Issue*, was first published in 1978. Before that, however, Thelma Wayler founded Green Mountain at Fox Run in Vermont as a non-diet retreat for women struggling with eating and weight. Her understanding of the issue began via her work in the 1950s, seeing the effects of restricted eating in children with diabetes. Also in the early 1970s, Carol Munter and Jane Hirschmann began Overcoming Overeating workshops in New York City, and eventually published a book by that name. Susie Orbach was a participant in Munter & Hirschmann's workshops. Geneen Roth's first book on emotional eating, "Feeding the Hungry Heart", was published in 1982. All identified conventional weight loss diets as the problem, and recommended intuitive eating (also called "attuned eating" or "the non-diet approach") as the solution. There also have been religious approaches to intuitive eating. Gwen Shamblin founded The Weigh Down Workshop in 1986. Thin Within workshops were started in 1975 by Judy Wardell-Halliday and Joy Imboden Overstreet. However, the book Thin Within published in 1985 had few, if any, religious overtones.

Evelyn Tribole and Elyse Resch coined the name in their 1995 book, *Intuitive Eating,* which outlines how to let go of dieting and become an intuitive eater. The first professional book on implementing this internally regulated eating, *Moving Away From Diets,* was written in 1996 by Karin Kratina, Nancy King and Dayle Hayes.

An early promoter in the recent wave of interest in intuitive eating is Lynn Donovan. She published a 1971 book called *The Anti-Diet: the pleasure power way to lose weight.*

Intuitive Eating Studies

In 2005, researcher Linda Bacon published the first two-year-long study demonstrating the effectiveness of Intuitive Eating. Later that year, Steven Hawks, a professor of Community Health at Brigham Young University, made headlines when he claimed to have lost 50 pounds following his version of an intuitive eating program. Hawks claims the underlying philosophies of intuitive eating are thousands of years old and exist in most eastern and some western religions. Intuitive eating is designed to be a "common sense, hunger-based approach to eating," where participants are encouraged to eat when and only when their body tells them it is hungry.

In 2006, Ohio State University researcher, Tracy Tylka, published a study which accomplished two key outcomes. First, Tylka developed and validated an assessment scale to define key traits of Intuitive Eaters, which are: unconditional permission to eat, eating for physical rather than emotional reasons, and reliance on internal hunger/satiety cues. Lastly, Tylka used that assessment scale on over 1400 people and determined that intuitive eaters have a higher sense of well being and lower body weights, without internalizing the "thin ideal".

Currently, University of Notre Dame psychology researcher, Lora Smitham, is recruiting people with binge eating disorder to study the effectiveness of the intuitive eating process for treating this problem. Smitham's premise is that dieting triggers binge eating and learning to become an intuitive eater can be therapeutic.

Maudsley Family Therapy

Maudsley family therapy also known as family-based treatment or Maudsley approach, is a family therapy for the treatment of anorexia nervosa devised by Christopher Dare and colleagues at the Maudsley Hospital in London. A comparison of family to individual therapy was conducted with eighty anorexia patients. The study showed family therapy to be the more effective approach in patients under 18 and within 3 years of the onset of their illness. Subsequent research confirmed the efficacy of family-based treatment for teens with anorexia nervosa. Family-based treatment has been adapted for bulimia nervosa and showed promising results in a randomized controlled trial comparing it to supportive individual therapy.

Maudsley Family Therapy is an evidenced-based approach to the treatment of anorexia nervosa and bulimia nervosa whose efficacy has been supported by empirical research.

Phases of Treatment

There are three phases involved in the Maudsley method, the treatment usually lasts one year and involves between 15-20 sessions. Daniel Le Grange, PhD and James Lock, MD, PhD describe the treatment as follows:

"The Maudsley approach can mostly be construed as an intensive outpatient treatment where parents play an active and positive role in order to: Help restore their child's weight to normal levels expected given their adolescent's age and height; hand the control over eating back to the adolescent, and; encourage normal adolescent development through an in-depth discussion of these crucial developmental issues as they pertain to their child.

More 'traditional' treatment of AN suggests that the clinician's efforts should be individually based. Strict adherents to the perspective of only individual treatment will insist that the participation of parents, whatever the format, is at best unnecessary, but worse still interference in the recovery process. In fact, many proponents of this approach would consider 'family problems' as part of the etiology of the AN. No doubt, this view might contribute to parents feeling themselves to blame for their child's illness. The Maudsley Approach opposes the notion that families are pathological or should be blamed for the development of AN. On the contrary, the Maudsley Approach considers the parents as a resource and essential in successful treatment for AN.

Phase I: Weight Restoration

The Maudsley Approach proceeds through three clearly defined phases, and is usually conducted within 15-20 treatment sessions over a period of about 12 months. In Phase I, also referred to as the weight restoration phase, the therapist focuses on the dangers of severe malnutrition associated with AN, such as hypothermia, growth hormone changes, cardiac dysfunction, and cognitive and emotional changes to name but a few, assessing the family's typical interaction pattern and eating habits, and assisting parents in re-feeding their daughter or son. The therapist will make every effort to help the parents in their joint attempt to restore their adolescent's weight. At the same time, the therapist will endeavor to align the patient with her/his siblings. A family meal is typically conducted during this phase, which serves at least two functions: It allows the therapist to observe the family's typical interaction patterns around eating, and it provides the therapist with an opportunity to assist the parents in their endeavor to encourage their adolescent to eat a little more than she was prepared to.

The way in which the parents go about this difficult but delicate task does not differ much in terms of the key principles and steps that a competent inpatient nursing team would follow. That is, an expression of sympathy and understanding by the parents with their adolescent's predicament of being ambivalent about this debilitating eating disorder, while at the same time being verbally persistent in their expectation that starvation is not an option. Most of this first phase of treatment is taken up by coaching the parents toward success in the weight restoration of their offspring, expressing support and empathy toward the adolescent given her dire predicament of entanglement with the illness, and realigning her with her siblings and peers. Realignment with one's siblings or peers means helping the adolescent to form stronger and more age appropriate relationships as opposed to being 'taken up' into a parental relationship.

Throughout, the role of the therapist is to model to the parents an uncritical stance toward the adolescent – the Maudsley Approach adheres to the tenet that the adolescent is not to blame for the challenging eating disorder behaviors, but rather that these symptoms are mostly outside of the adolescent's control (externalizing the illness). At no point should this phase of treatment be interpreted as a 'green light' for parents to be critical of their child. Quite the contrary, the therapist will work hard to address any parental criticism or hostility toward the adolescent.

Phase II: Returning Control over Eating to the Adolescent

The patient's acceptance of parental demand for increased food intake, steady weight gain, as well as a change in the mood of the family (i.e., relief at having taken charge of the eating disorder), all signal the start of Phase II of treatment.

This phase of treatment focuses on encouraging the parents to help their child to take more control over eating once again. The therapist advises the parents to accept that the main task here is the return of their child to physical health, and that this now happens mostly in a way that is in keeping with their child's age and their parenting style. Although symptoms remain central in the discussions between the therapist and the family, weight gain with minimum tension is encouraged. In addition, all other general family relationship issues or difficulties in terms of day-to-day adolescent or parenting concerns that the family has had to postpone can now be brought forward for review. This, however, occurs only in relationship to the effect these issues have on the parents in their task of assuring steady weight gain. For example, the patient may want to go out with her friends to have dinner and a movie. However, while the parents are still unsure whether their child would eat entirely on her own accord, she might be required to have dinner with her parents and then be allowed to join friends for a movie.

Phase III: Establishing Healthy Adolescent Identity

Phase III is initiated when the adolescent is able to maintain weight above 95% of ideal weight on her/his own and self-starvation has abated.

Treatment focus starts to shift to the impact AN has had on the individual establishing a healthy adolescent identity. This entails a review of central issues of adolescence and includes supporting increased personal autonomy for the adolescent, the development of appropriate parental boundaries, as well as the need for the parents to reorganize their life together after their children's prospective departure."

Evidence-based Strategy

To date there have been 4 randomized controlled trials of Maudsley Family Therapy. The first (Russell et al., 1987) compared the Maudsley Model to individual therapy and found that family-based treatment was more effective for patients under 19 years of age with less than three years duration of illness. Ninety percent of these patients achieved a normal weight or the return of menses at the end of treatment including at 5 year follow-up (Eisler, et al., 1997).Two further randomised trials compared standard Maudsley treatment with a modified version where the patients and parents were seen separately (Le Grange et al. 1992, Eisler et al., 2000). In these trials approximately 70% of patients returned to a normal body weight (>90% IBW) or experienced the return of menses at the end of treatment, regardless of which version of the model was employed. Results from a more recent randomised controlled trial suggest that results are maintained with the manualisation of the Maudsley approach (Lock & Le Grange, 2001). There is also evidence that a short (6 months) and a long course (1 year) of treatment results in a similar positive outcome (Lock et al., 2005). Finally, the outcome using family-based treatment appears just as positive for children (9–12 years old) as it does for adolescents (Lock et al., 2006).

References

- Shapiro, Jennifer R. (2010). "Mobile therapy: Use of text-messaging in the treatment of bulimia nervosa". International Journal of Eating Disorders. 43 (6): 513–519. doi:10.1002/eat.20744

- Fairburn, Christopher G. (2008). Cognitive behavior therapy and eating disorders. New York: Guilford Press. ISBN 1593857098

- Groves, PhD, Barry (2002). "WILLIAM BANTING: The Father of the Low-Carbohydrate Diet". Second Opinions. Retrieved 26 December 2007

- Strychar I (January 2006). "Diet in the management of weight loss". CMAJ. 174 (1): 56–63. PMC 1319349. PMID 16389240. doi:10.1503/cmaj.045037

- Kross, E., Bruehlman-Senecal, E., Park, J., Burson, A., Dougherty, A., Shablack, H., & Ayduk, O. (2014). Self-talk as a regulatory mechanism: How you do it matters. Journal of personality and social psychology, 106(2), 304

- O'Neil, William J. (2003). Business Leaders & Success: 55 Top Business Leaders & How They Achieved Greatness. McGraw-Hill Professional. pp. 35–36. ISBN 0-07-142680-9

- Halton TL, Willett WC, Liu S, et al. (2006). "Low-carbohydrate-diet score and the risk of coronary heart disease in women". N. Engl. J. Med. 355 (19): 1991–2002. PMID 17093250. doi:10.1056/NEJMoa055317

- Priebe, Stefan; Wright, Donna (2006). "The provision of psychotherapy – An international comparison". Journal of Public Mental Health. 5 (3): 12–22 (16). doi:10.1108/17465729200600022

- Buckley, C (1998). God Is My Broker, A Monk-Tycoon Reveals the 7 1/2 Laws of Spiritual and Financial Growth. Random House. pp. Page 185. ISBN 0-06-097761-2

- "Arrêté du 9 juin 2010 relatif aux demandes d'inscription au registre national des psychothérapeutes" (in French). Retrieved 21 July 2010

- McGivern, Gerry; Fischer, Michael Daniel (2012). "Reactivity and reactions to regulatory transparency in medicine, psychotherapy and counselling". Social Science & Medicine. 74 (3): 289–96. PMID 22104085. doi:10.1016/j.socscimed.2011.09.035

- Carlson E., Dain N (1960). "The Psychotherapy that was Moral Treatment". The American Journal of Psychiatry. 117 (6): 519–524. doi:10.1176/ajp.117.6.519

- Skipper, Annalynn (2009-10-07). Advanced Medical Nutrition Therapy Practice. Jones & Bartlett Learning. p. 50. ISBN 9780763742898

- "The top 10: The most influential therapists of the past quarter-century". Psychotherapy Networker. March–April 2007. Archived from the original on 5 February 2011. Retrieved 7 October 2010

- Markowitz JC1 Weissman MM (Mar 2012). "Interpersonal psychotherapy: past, present and future". Clin Psychol Psychother. 19 (2): 99–105. PMC 3427027. PMID 22331561. doi:10.1002/cpp.1774

- Corp, Nadia; Tsaroucha, Anna; Kingston, Paul (2008). "Human givens therapy: The evidence base". Mental Health Review Journal. 13 (4): 44–52. doi:10.1108/13619322200800027

- Kawash, Samira (2013). Candy: A Century of Panic and Pleasure. New York: Faber & Faber, Incorporated. pp. 185–189. ISBN 9780865477568

- Wierzbicki, Michael; Pekarik, Gene (1993). "A meta-analysis of psychotherapy dropout". Professional Psychology: Research and Practice. 24 (2): 190–5. doi:10.1037/0735-7028.24.2.190

- Welling, Hans (June 2012). "Transformative emotional sequence: towards a common principle of change" (PDF). Journal of Psychotherapy Integration. 22 (2): 109–136. doi:10.1037/a0027786

Permissions

Index